Working in international health

SUCCESS IN MEDICINE SERIES

Working in international health

WRITTEN BY

Maïa Gedde
Programme Manager, SURF Rwanda

Susana Edjang
Programme Manager, Zambia UK Health Workforce Alliance

Kate Mandeville
Specialist Registrar in Public Health and Wellcome Trust
Research Fellow, London School of Hygiene and Tropical Medicine

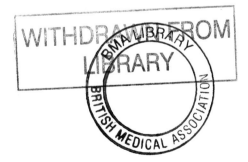

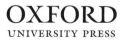

OXFORD
UNIVERSITY PRESS

OXFORD

UNIVERSITY PRESS

Great Clarendon Street, Oxford ox2 6DP

Oxford University Press is a department of the University of Oxford.
It furthers the University's objective of excellence in research, scholarship,
and education by publishing worldwide in

Oxford New York

Auckland Cape Town Dar es Salaam Hong Kong Karachi
Kuala Lumpur Madrid Melbourne Mexico City Nairobi
New Delhi Shanghai Taipei Toronto

With offices in

Argentina Austria Brazil Chile Czech Republic France Greece
Guatemala Hungary Italy Japan Poland Portugal Singapore
South Korea Switzerland Thailand Turkey Ukraine Vietnam

Oxford is a registered trade mark of Oxford University Press
in the UK and in certain other countries

Published in the United States
by Oxford University Press Inc., New York

British Library Cataloguing in Publication Data
Data available

Library of Congress Cataloging in Publication Data
Data available

Typeset in Charter by Cenveo, Bangalore, India
Printed and bound by
CPI Group (UK) Ltd, Croydon, CR0 4YY

ISBN 978–0–19–960071–7

10 9 8 7 6 5 4 3 2 1

To my parents, JP and the one to be (MG)
To my mother, Teresa-Adjiri (SE)
To my husband for all his support (KM)

Acknowledgements

We are extremely indebted to our editors at OUP, Christopher Reid and Katy Loftus, for making this book possible and for their support along the way. Also to our anonymous OUP reviewers who were very diligent and provided valuable comments on the draft chapters.

We would also like to acknowledge the contribution of the following people for the role they played in shaping this book, whether they agreed to be interviewed by us, contributed to case studies, helped us with information or reviewed sections of the book. The book is much richer thanks to their experiences. The list is long so we apologise if we have unknowingly omitted anyone.

Aisha Dodwell (MSF), Alice Cannon, Alex Talbot (Operation Smile), Alison Herbert, Amina Aitsi-Selmi, Andrew Lee, Androula Ozcivi (RCN), Anne Fuller, Arantza Faiges-Hijon, Beth Cheeseborough, Bill Bavington, Bill Clucas, Bjarne Garden (NORAD), Brenda Longstaff (Northumbria Healthcare NHS FT), Catherine Allum (DOW), Carlos Martin-Saborido, Charlie Easmon, Chris Lavy, Christine Hancock, Colin Beckworth, Colin Green, Conchi Martin Cortijo, Conall Watson, Damien Awog-Boro, David Ross, David Parry, Delan Devakumar, Dele Fatunla, Dianne Pickering, Edmond Baganzi, Eldryd Parry (THET), Emma Richards, Enyi Anosike (Nigeria Public Health Network), Erica Mitchell (British Red Cross), Fleur Kitsell (NHS South Central), Francis Kangata, Geraldine Kelly, Graeme Chisholm (VSO), Gwyneth Lewis, Helen Asquith, Ines Smyth (Oxfam), Jane Fitzpatrick, Janet Kerrigan, Jay Bagaria (DH), Jean Bailey, Jean Claude Mugunga, Jean-Marc Jacobs (MSF), Jed Boardman, Jennifer Hall, Jim Campbell (Integrare), Jim Easton (NHS South Central), Joanna Manson, John MacDermot, Jonathan Fitzsimon, Katie Wakeham, Kenneth Barrand, Ken Levere, Kevin Marsh (KEMRI-Wellcome), Kielan Yarrow, Lesley Dawson, Liz Crawford (MSF), Liz Ollier, Lois Boyle, Lola Banjoko, Louise Blanks, Lucy-Anna Kelly, Lucy Reynolds, Lydia Stone, Marielle Connan, Mark Roberts, Mark Snelling (Interhealth), Mark Whyman, Marko Kerac, Maryann Noronha, Matthew Harris, Michael Pelly, Michael Roe, Mike Rowson (UCL), Murray Cochrane (NHS International Group), Mwayi Madanitsa, Najeeb Rahman (Doctors Worldwide), Nick Banatvala (WHO), Nicola Wales, Nic Scarborough (RedR), Noemi Diaz Matas, Ollie Ross, Pamela Dzalah, Paulina Keinanen (Skillshare), Petronella Mwasandube, Phil McDonald, Philippa Cornish (British Red Cross), Pia McRae (THET), Rachel Isaac, Rachel Jenkins, Raúl Pardíñaz-Solís, Remy Serge Manzi, Richard Dowden (RAS), Rob Aldridge, Rob Delacour, Rob Stewart, Ruth Grearson (VSO), Ruth Rottbeck, Shazia Ovaisi, Sian Crisp, Simon Little, Stephen Flannagan, Stephen Hitchin, Sudeep Chand, Sue and Martin McCaig, Sue Jacob, Tana Wuliji, Tiwonge Khonje, Tom Lissauer, Valerie Powell, Vicky Lavy, Will Snell, William Buckland, Zahida Ahmad, Zoe Anne Walker.

We would also like to thank Angel Edjang Mangue for his excellent work on the illustrations and Thomas J. Harte for producing the superb regional maps in Chapter 6.

Whilst we have kept the majority of our case studies anonymous, we have used names with permission where appropriate.

Foreword by Lord Nigel Crisp

For many years health workers from the UK have travelled abroad to help improve health care in other countries and to learn and develop their own skills. This book provides an invaluable guide to how to so most effectively.

It is a very practical book which deals with the preparation that is needed and provides ideas about how to avoid common problems as well as offering a very good analysis of the wider context of health globally which forms the backdrop to any visit. Crucially, it also describes how to learn about the culture of the country and respect the local traditions and customs—and avoid the all too common trap of assuming that our ways are the best and that we can simply use our own tried and tested solutions to equally good effect in a new context.

In recent years pioneers such as Sir Eldryd Parry of the Tropical Health Education Trust (THET) have provided leadership and support for developing partnerships—links and twining arrangements - between organisations in different parts of the world which help provide continuity and an institutional framework for personal links and relationships across the continents.

Most recently the Welsh, Scottish and UK Governments have all responded with, amongst other things, a UK strategy *"Health is Global"* and a response to my own report *"Global Health Partnerships"* - both of which acknowledge the value to the UK and other countries from partnerships and exchange between health workers and institutions and the individual experience of working in another country and another environment. In 2010 the Government announced the creation of a £20 million fund over 4 years to support such partnerships.

Progress is being made but needs to go further. Once again pioneers, including the authors of this book, are showing what needs to be done to make experience of working in other health systems not just acceptable but a vital part of the education and development of good health workers in the UK and elsewhere.

The simple truth is that UK health workers can contribute an enormous amount to improving health in low and middle income countries; just as many health workers from those countries have contributed to the NHS. At the same time they can learn and develop new skills. It should be no surprise that much can be learned from people who without our resources and the baggage of our history are creating new ideas and innovating in ways we can learn from.

Knowledge transfer is two way. Everyone has something to teach and everyone has something to learn.

Nigel Crisp is an Independent Crossbench member of the House of Lords. He was Chief Executive of the NHS in England and Permanent Secretary of the Department of Health from 2000 to 2006. His book *Turning the World Upside Down—the search for global health in the 21st Century* was published in 2010.

Foreword by
Professor Parveen Kumar

International and Global Health are now on the agenda for every healthcare professional and students of the health professions. Many ask enthusiastically of how they can get involved but, when they do get the chance, they are quite unprepared and unaware of what is really required of them. Enthusiasm is clearly not enough and here is where this book is an absolute 'must'!

'*Working in international health*' is a comprehensive resource and covers all the questions that health workers and students will ask on going abroad. It describes the step by step process of how to plan and undertake a placement. Practical details and hurdles that need to be addressed are given so that aspiring workers can actually use their time effectively and efficiently. It will certainly provide the confidence to do the job well and ensure one is not a hindrance to those in the field. The chapters take the reader from firstly asking the pertinent question of whether 'international work is for me' (very important to the future outcome of a placement) through to coming home, where many may need extra help to re-acclimatise to life back home. They also recognise the importance of not only debriefing but also in the dissemination and sharing of what has been learnt. It is not all easy going and this book will help you recognise the moods that you might go through from your first few days of anticipation and exhilaration to discouragement, irritability, restlessness and finally finding equilibrium in your working day.

What I really liked about this book is that the message is always set out on a background of data, evidence and practical information. Global health and disease statistics are given along with information on what has worked and what, sadly, has not! A lesson for not repeating expensive ventures but also a lesson that gives us the understanding of what is required at the local level. It is not about what 'I can do for them' but 'what do they want me to help them do with them'!

The book gives illustrations of real peoples' careers combining work in the UK with time overseas. These include careers of medical students, trainees, consultants, nurses, pharmacists and others, and these examples provide helpful points for all. They give an insight into what might be expected of you to retain and keep up with colleagues at home, so that you are not compromised in your promotion on return from abroad.

The authors are all experts and bring with them an enormous background of practical experience in many countries. They complement each other extremely well in their knowledge and provide information from their own careers in management, health economics, international development, physiotherapy and public health. I would highly recommend this book as a handbook for all studying global health modules or going abroad to work in the healthcare field.

Parveen Kumar CBE, BSc, MD, FRCP, FRCPE
Professor of Medicine and Education
Barts and the London School of Medicine and Dentistry
Queen Mary, University of London

Introduction

When people hear that we are involved in international health work, their eyes light up. 'Oh, I've been thinking about taking 6 months off to volunteer overseas,' says the nurse in the GP practice. 'It's something I want to do after I retire, what would you suggest?' asks the surgeon we meet at the international health conference. And an e-mail arrives in from a medical student wanting contacts in Nepal to help plan her elective.

Working overseas in low and middle-income countries (LMIC) is what many of the more adventurous UK health professionals aspire to. It provides an opportunity to share your skills with those in the greatest need and can remind you of the reason you chose a health profession in the first place. Global health has become an increasingly popular course amongst the younger generations. Newly qualified professionals are taking advantage of few commitments to go overseas for a year or two. And senior professionals would like to share their skills in places and crises publicised by the global media.

Yet despite this interest and enthusiasm among UK health professionals, we couldn't find one comprehensive resource that would cover the many questions about making international health a reality in their lives. So we set about writing one.

This book is aimed at all health professionals interested in international health work. It may be something you've been thinking about for a while, but haven't acted on yet. When is the best point to take time out? Perhaps you are a student who wants the opportunity to work and travel or even an international career. How can you gear your qualifications and experience towards this? You may even have done some international work already, but want to continue to be engaged from the UK. What opportunities exist?

But we have tried to go beyond the simple what, where and when questions. How do you know which is the best organisation to fit your needs? Why is it important to align your work with local priorities to ensure your efforts have a long-lasting impact? What are the challenges of working in a resource-poor environment? And how can you ensure your time overseas enhances your career upon your return?

Whilst we have a solid understanding of these issues between us, this is far from comprehensive. So throughout the book we have sought the ideas, opinions and sage advice from experienced professionals, enabling us to share their experiences with you.

It has been an interesting book to write, allowing us to explore in depth the issues that we have encountered on a daily basis in our work, and seeking thoughts and opinions from both those who are experts and novices in the field. We hope you find it equally interesting to read.

Who this guide is for

This guide is for all UK health workers who are interested in working in international health. Whether you are planning your first foray overseas, or you already have some experience and are looking for more, this book is aimed at you.

At this point you might be wondering what the distinction is between international health and global health. Why have we not called this book 'Working in Global Health'? It can be confusing. Global health focuses on issues that directly or indirectly affect health and can transcend national boundaries. Its major objective is to achieve health equity among nations and for all people. Development and implementation of solutions often requires global cooperation. So if you are working for a multilateral organisation, such as the United Nations (UN), you may be involved in global health.

International health in contrast focuses on the health issues of countries other than one's own, especially those of LMIC. It seeks to help people of other nations, and the development and implementation of solutions usually requires bi-national cooperation. So both terms are used in this book, but we use international health to describe the kind of work overseas that you're probably interested in.

Following on from that, overseas in this book refers to only LMIC (sometimes referred to as developing or second/third-world countries). Although many UK health professionals work overseas in high-income countries like Australia and New Zealand, this is not the focus of international health and specific guidance is available elsewhere.

Although this book is within the Success in Medicine series, it features advice and case studies from a whole range of health professionals, working in service delivery or academia, including: doctors, nurses, midwives, pharmacists, physiotherapists, clinical psychologists, paramedics and managers. All kinds of health professionals are able to make a contribution overseas.

Most of the information in this book is generic and is useful for all health workers. Where there is profession-specific guidance available, we have included it. Unfortunately, this is currently limited outside medicine and nursing. With more and more UK health workers engaging in international work, we hope that by the next edition there will be detailed guidance available for more professions.

REFERENCE

Koplan JP (2009). Towards a common definition of global health. *Lancet* 373: 1993–5.

How to use this guide

If your current knowledge of international health is minimal, the book takes you through a step-by-step process of considering, planning and undertaking a placement. If you feel this is you, then we would advise you to read at least the first two sections in order, as this will help you understand the opportunities within international health.

Those with more experience, on the other hand, may want to dip in and out of the book as interest takes them. For some topics, we cross-refer to other chapters, where these issues are explained more fully.

Whether expert or novice, you will find it useful to take the book with you when you do go abroad, as there are parts that will help you to think through your time overseas and are useful to reread if you encounter difficulties. Please do get in contact to share any relevant experiences with us, which will help improve future editions.

The four sections as a whole lead you through a period of international work, from starting out through to your return home and beyond. **Section 1 (Is international work for me?)** puts this type of work into perspective, and helps you assess if it's possible for you right now. If you decide the time is right, **Section 2 (Making it happen)** is a very practical guide to choosing what work to do, and where and with whom to do it. Once you've arrived at your destination, **Section 3 (In the field)** gives you an honest insight into life overseas. Although you'll probably skim through these chapters before you go, try to read them more deeply whilst you are there for further guidance and reassurance. Finally, **Section 4 (Coming home)** steers you through the process of re-immersion into UK life and work, and how to continue your involvement in international health.

Authors' biographies

Maïa Gedde is an international development professional with experience of programme management and institutional capacity building in the health, education and employment sectors. While at the Tropical Health and Education Trust (THET) she helped to develop, coordinate and evaluate health partnerships between the National Health Service (NHS) and hospitals and training institutions in Malawi, Ghana and Uganda. She wrote the first and second editions of *The International Health Links Manual: A Guide to Starting up and Maintaining Long Term Health Partnerships*. She currently lives between Rwanda and Morocco.

Susana Edjang helped set up and runs the Zambia UK Health Workforce Alliance, a network of Zambia- and UK-based organisations supporting health initiatives in Zambia. She is also a researcher and advisor on global health and climate change at the UK's House of Lords. Prior to this, she was Health Links Manager at the THET where she helped the strategy, growth and recognition of the Health Links' movement in the UK and promoted Health Links across UK, African and Asian health and development organisations. Susana trained as a physiotherapist and a development economist.

Kate Mandeville is a public health doctor based in London, UK. She was born in Malawi and grew up in Nepal. She has experience of clinical practice, project management, and research in several sub-Saharan African countries. Whilst a junior doctor, she set up Medic to Medic, a charity supporting trainee health workers in low-income countries. She is currently based at the London School of Hygiene and Tropical Medicine (LSHTM), researching her PhD into the cost-effectiveness of incentives for health workers.

Abbreviations

AIDS	acquired immunodeficiency syndrome
BMA	British Medical Association
BMJ	British Medical Journal
BRC	British Red Cross
CCST	Certificate of Completion of Specialist Training
CDC	Centers for Disease Control and Prevention
CMF	Christian Medical Fellowship
CMR	crude mortality rate
CPD	continuing professional development
CRS	Catholic Relief Service
DALY	Disability-Adjusted Life Year
DFID	Department for International Development
DH	Department of Health, UK
DOW	Doctors of the World
DWW	Doctors Worldwide
EEA	European Economic Area
ENT	Ear, Nose and Throat
EU	European Union
FBO	Faith-Based Organisations
FCO	Foreign and Commonwealth Office
GMC	General Medical Council
GMF	Global Medical Force
GP	General Practitioner
GPI	Global Peace Index
HAP	Humanitarian Accountability Partnership
HCHA	high child mortality, high adult mortality
HCVHA	high child mortality, very high adult mortality
HIV	human immunodeficiency virus
HMRC	Her Majesty's Revenue and Customs
HR	human resources
HRH	Human Resources for Health
ICRC	International Committee of the Red Cross

IFRC	International Federation of Red Cross and Red Crescent Societies
IHL	International Humanitarian Law
IHLC	International Health Links Centre
IHP	International Health Partnership
LATH	Liverpool Associates in Tropical Health
LCLA	low child mortality, low adult mortality
LMIC	low and middle-income countries
LSHTM	London School of Hygiene and Tropical Medicine
LSTM	Liverpool School of Tropical Medicine
MDDUS	Medical and Dental Defence Union of Scotland
MDG	Millennium Development Goal
MDU	Medical Defence Union
MPS	Medical Protection Society
MSE	Medical Student Electives
MSF	Médecins sans Frontières
MTAS	Medical Training Application Service
NGO	non-governmental organisation
NHS	National Health Service
OCO	orthopaedic clinical officer
ODA	Overseas Development Agency
OECD	Organisation for Economic Co-operation and Development
OOP	out of programme (time out of specialist training programmes)
OOPC	out of programme (career break)
OOPE	out of programme (experience)
OOPR	out of programme (research)
OOPT	out of programme (training)
PDP	personal development plan
PEP	post-exposure prophylaxis
PEPFAR	(United States) President's Emergency Plan for AIDS Relief
PPP	Public Private Partnerships
PSF	Pharmacists Without Borders
R&R	rest and recuperation
RCM	Royal College of Midwives
RCN	Royal College of Nursing
RCPCH	Royal College of Paediatrics and Child Health
SLC	Student Loans Company
SWAp	Sector Wide Approach
THET	Tropical Health and Education Trust
TB	Tuberculosis

ToT	training of trainers
UK	United Kingdom
UN	United Nations
UNDP	United Nations Development Programme
UNV	United Nations Volunteers
USD	United States Dollars
VLCLA	very low child mortality, low adult mortality
VSO	Voluntary Service Overseas
WHO	World Health Organization

Contents

Appendices

Is international work for me?

Every day thousands of people die unnecessarily from preventable diseases; diseases we know how to cure and regularly do in rich countries. In one corner of the world, a team of health professionals spends hours on a cosmetic surgery procedure. In another a newborn baby and its mother die because there are no qualified health workers in the vicinity to attend a complicated birth. Health and healthcare are far from equally distributed around the world.

But you may be able to contribute towards changing this. This first section of the book examines the complex world of global health and what your role might be in this.

Chapter 1 (A global perspective) provides an overview of health in the world today, and looks at some of the major reasons for health inequalities. What have been the global and the UK's responses to these issues?

Chapter 2 (Why do it?) focuses on you as an individual wanting to play a role in international health. It looks at common motivations for wanting to go overseas and how to balance these to manage your expectations.

Chapter 3 (Rewards and challenges) looks at the pros and cons for you, the host country and the bigger picture. It will give you a flavour of what you can gain but also the realities of this type of work.

And finally, **Chapter 4 (Is it possible?)** helps you to evaluate whether international work is right for you at this stage of your life. It provides some practical steps about how you can combine international work with a UK career and includes examples of how others have managed to combine the two.

Having read through this section, you will have a better idea of whether this type of work is for you and where, as one individual, you fit into the global context. If you have already had some experience of working internationally, it may help you to reflect on whether you want to continue working in this area, perhaps even making a career out of it. The next section then takes you through the specifics of arranging your time abroad.

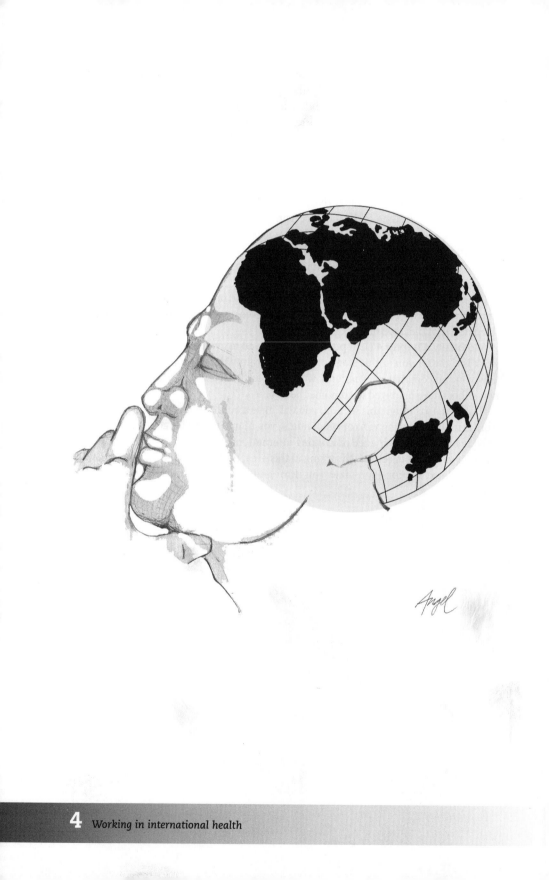

CHAPTER 1

The global perspective

What is happening out there? Who is doing what in international health? You may have heard terms like the Millennium Development Goals (MDGs), Global Fund and bilateral aid bandied around. What do they mean exactly? How do they relate to each other and what impact, if any, will they have on your work overseas?

Welcome to the global health jigsaw puzzle. This chapter gives you an overview of how all the pieces fit together. The first part introduces some of the key issues in global health. We then look at how the world is responding to these challenges and why strong health systems are crucial. The final section examines the UK's response and where you might fit into the jigsaw.

This chapter is necessarily broad in focus, but do follow up on the references provided to delve deeper into these issues.

Health in a poor environment

It is easy to become complacent about health when we live in a country where health-care is available from the cradle to the grave, and based on clinical need rather than the ability to pay. This type of healthcare makes us incredibly fortunate compared to the majority of the world's population.

If you had been born in a poor country, surviving childhood would have been one of the greatest achievements of your life [one in eight children in Sub-Saharan Africa die before their fifth birthday (UN 2010)]. As for your mother, she risked her life giving birth to you [99% of maternal deaths occur in low and middle-income countries (LMIC) (WHO 2010)]. As you grow up, you experience love and relationships in an environment where up to one in four of your friends have HIV (UNAIDS 2010). If you fall ill, you may have to travel many kilometres to find a health clinic. When you get to the hospital, the staff may not see you unless you have the money to pay up front [worldwide it is estimated that 100 million people every year are pushed into poverty by healthcare costs (Rowson 2007)]. And after all that, you might not receive the correct treatment, as the drugs have run out or a lack of equipment or skills has led to the wrong diagnosis.

Health inequalities around the world

Billions of people do not have access to free or subsidised healthcare, trained or sufficient health workers and effective or cheap medicines. For instance:

- Sub-Saharan Africa has 11% of the world's population and 25% of the global burden of disease, but only 3% of the global health workforce and less than 1% of the global health expenditure (WHO 2006).
- Only 20% of the global expenditure of medicines is spent in Africa, Asia, the Middle East and Latin America with 80% of the population and 92% of the disease burden (Global Health Watch 2005).
- It is estimated that about 10% of the world's medical research is devoted to conditions that account for 90% of the global disease burden. This is known as the 10/90 gap (Global Forum for Health Research 2011).

Although the picture may seem bleak, there have been some notable successes in global health over the past few decades. Table 1.1 lists some of these successes alongside some of today's sad realities. It's important to be aware of the successes as they remind us of what is possible. The failures need not be inevitable and can indicate where to focus efforts for improvements.

Find out more

Levine R (2007) *Case Studies in Global Health: Millions Saved*. Centre for Global Development. *http://www.cgdev.org*
    This book describes 20 case studies in which large-scale efforts to improve health in poor countries have succeeded—saving millions of lives. It provides clear evidence that global health challenges which are often perceived as daunting are indeed solvable, and suggests how successes can be achieved in the future.

What still kills?

The principal causes of death in LMIC are respiratory infections, HIV/AIDS, perinatal infections, diarrhoeal disease and tropical diseases such as malaria. This pattern of disease—where infectious diseases are much more common than other diseases—is

Table 1.1 Successes and failures in global health

The good: successes in global health	The bad: failures in global health
• Measles deaths in the African region have been reduced by 90% from 2000 to 2008, through disease control and mass vaccination campaigns (CDC 2009).	• Seventeen children under the age of 5 die every minute; 70% of these deaths are preventable (UN 2010).
• A multi-agency strategy to control onchocerciasis (river blindness) in Sub-Saharan Africa has allowed 22 million children in 11 countries to be free of the threat of blindness (Levine 2007).	• One woman will die for every 100 live births or less in the worst-off countries (WHO 2010).
• The prevalence of tuberculosis (TB) in China has been reduced by 40% between 1990 and 2000 through the introduction of directly observed treatment (Levine 2007).	• An estimated 26% of the adult population in Swaziland has HIV/AIDS (UNAIDS 2010).
• Contraceptive use in Bangladesh has increased from 3% to 64% (with a decrease in fertility from seven to three children per woman) through a robust outreach approach over three decades (Levine 2007).	• Ten countries in Sub-Saharan Africa have fewer than three doctors per 100,000 people. The global average is 146 per 100,000 (WHO 2006).
	• Government spending on health varies from just $36 per person in South East Asia to $1401 in Europe (WHO 2010).

very similar to that of Britain 100 years ago. In 1880 infectious diseases accounted for at least 33% of deaths in the UK. In 1997 this figure had fallen to 17% (Hicks and Allen 1999).

As countries develop, sanitation and preventative healthcare such as vaccination tend to shift the major causes of death from communicable diseases towards those associated with longer life expectancy such as cancer and heart disease. However, some countries such as India and South Africa are now suffering a double burden of disease: where a continued high burden of communicable disease co-exists with increasing risk factors for non-communicable disease, particularly in urban settings. Often this burden is polarised by wealth: with richer communities at higher risk of chronic diseases and poorer communities still dying from infectious diseases.

However, measuring mortality alone can be misleading. The Disability-Adjusted Life Year (DALY), developed by the World Health Organization (WHO) is a measure to quantify the burden of disease from all causes including injuries and their risk factors. The DALY is based on years of life lost from premature death plus years of life lived in less than full health. Using DALYs reveals some surprising figures, for example that depression causes the third highest burden of disease in the world (see Table 2).

Table 1.2 Leading global causes of mortality and burden of disease, 2004

Rank	Mortality	%	DALYS	%
1	Ischaemic heart disease	12.2	Lower respiratory infections	6.2
2	Cerebrovascular disease	9.7	Diarrhoeal diseases	4.8
3	Lower respiratory infections	7.1	Depression	4.3
4	Chronic obstructive pulmonary disease	5.1	Ischaemic heart disease	4.1
5	Diarrhoeal diseases	3.7	HIV/AIDS	3.8
6	HIV/AIDS	3.5	Cerebrovascular disease	3.1
7	TB	2.5	Prematurity, low birth weight	2.9
8	Trachea, bronchus, lung cancers	2.3	Birth asphyxia, birth trauma	2.7
9	Road traffic accidents	2.2	Road traffic accidents	2.7
10	Prematurity, low birth weight	2	Neonatal infections and other	2.7

Source: WHO (2004) The Global Burden of Disease: 2004 update

Find out more

- The Global Burden of Disease Project: *http://www.who.int/healthinfo/global_burden_disease/about/en/index.html*
- World Health Report 2002—Reducing Risks, Promoting Healthy Life: *http://www.who.int/whr/2002/en/index.html*

The global response

There is a need to promote more equitable access to health and healthcare around the world. Preventing avoidable deaths in an age of plenty is a moral and humanitarian imperative. In addition, the extent of globalisation means that we can no longer consider the health of one country in isolation. This was never more obvious than during the 2009–10 H1N1 influenza (swine flu) pandemic. Governments are realising that global health issues must be addressed not only to help those directly affected, but also for the safety and security of their own citizens.

Governments of high, middle and low income countries are all playing their role (although some with more political will than others) in the response to global health issues, as are businesses, philanthropic groups, non-governmental organisations (NGOs), individuals and communities. This means that global health assistance is exceedingly complex. It has been estimated that there are 40 governments donating aid, 26 United Nation (UN) agencies, 20 global and regional funds and 90 global health initiatives all involved in global health policy (McColl 2008). These figures do not include the numerous NGOs and other partners working in this sector for which the numbers reach thousands. In order to be effective, these organisations need to work together. The Global Governance Monitor from the Council on International Relations has a directory of global health and finance organisations, outlining their history and current functions (http://www.cfr.org/healthmonitor).

What does the WHO do?

The WHO is the directing and coordinating authority for health within the UN system. It is responsible for providing leadership on global health matters, shaping the health research agenda, setting norms and standards, articulating evidence-based policy options, providing technical support to countries and monitoring and assessing health trends. The WHO has its headquarters in Geneva, six regional offices and 147 country and liaison offices.

Find out more

The World Health Report, first published in 1995, is WHO's leading publication. Produced annually, the report combines an expert assessment of global health, including statistics relating to all countries, with a focus on a specific subject. The main purpose of the report is to provide countries, donor agencies, international organisations and others with the information they need to help them make policy and funding decisions.

- *http://www.who.int/whr*

Coordination and financing are two key obstacles to achieving improved health care. The WHO Commission on Macroeconomics and Health laid the ground for scaling up domestic health financing which contributed to one of the single most important global initiatives so far. This is the commitment by 189 heads of state and major global health organisations to the MDGs. These were set in 2000 with a target date of 2015. Three of the eight MDGs are specifically related to health:

- MDG4: Reduce child mortality (by two thirds)
- MDG5: Improve maternal health (reducing by three quarters the maternal mortality ratio - i.e. the number of maternal deaths per 100,000 live births)
- MDG6: Combat HIV/AIDS, malaria and other diseases

Some argue that the MDGs are over-simplistic and focus on high mortality diseases, whilst ignoring those that cause high morbidity, such as mental health and neglected tropical diseases. This may be true, but the MDGs also brought with them the realisation that vertical programmes (those that focus on single diseases or conditions) were limited in their approach, because weak health systems hindered their success. This changed the focus to strengthening health systems as a whole (the so-called horizontal programmes).

Find out more

Despite the MDGs and increasing political interest in global health, overseas aid spending specifically on health still falls short of what is needed. The organisation Action for Global Health provides information about the way that Europe should be supporting LMIC to achieve the health MDG targets.

• *http://www.actionforglobalhealth.eu*

Health systems at the heart of good health

"A health system is the sum total of all the organizations, institutions and resources whose primary purpose is to improve health. A health system needs staff, funds, information, supplies, transport, communications and overall guidance and direction. And it needs to provide services that are responsive and financially fair, while treating people decently."

World Health Organization (http://www.who.int/topics/health_systems/qa/ en/index.html)

The realisation that vertical health programmes, which focus on a single disease, could distort local priorities to the detriment of the overall health of the population led to a refocus on health systems as the heart of good health. Figure 1.1 illustrates four important pillars to any health system, which include:

1 A good *health financing* system which raises adequate funds for health, in ways that ensure people can use needed services, and are protected from financial catastrophe or impoverishment associated with having to pay for them.

2 A well-performing *health workforce*. This needs to be sufficient in number with a mix of staff and skills, fairly distributed, competent, responsive and productive. ·

3 *Leadership and governance* which ensures a strategic policy framework exists that is combined with effective oversight, coalition-building, the provision of appropriate regulations and incentives, attention to system design and accountability.

4 A well-functioning *health information system* which ensures the production, analysis, dissemination and use of reliable and timely information on health determinants, health systems performance and health status to allow for effective planning.

The WHO has identified two other building blocks of health systems: equitable access to essential *medical products and technologies,* and effective *service delivery.* But efficient individual pillars will not solve the problem alone; the different pillars must work in synergy with each other for a well-functioning health system (http://www.who.int/healthsystems/en/). This requires a collaborative approach between international partners (Figure 1.1).

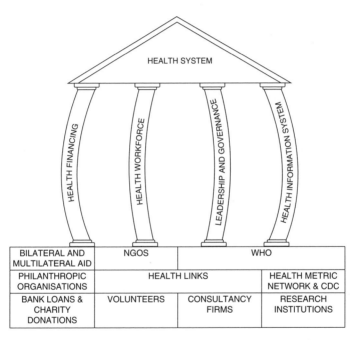

HEALTH SYSTEM

HEALTH FINANCING

HEALTH WORKFORCE

LEADERSHIP AND GOVERNANCE

HEALTH INFORMATION SYSTEM

BILATERAL AND MULTILATERAL AID	NGOS		WHO
PHILANTHROPIC ORGANISATIONS	HEALTH LINKS		HEALTH METRIC NETWORK & CDC
BANK LOANS & CHARITY DONATIONS	VOLUNTEERS	CONSULTANCY FIRMS	RESEARCH INSTITUTIONS

Figure 1.1 Four of the key pillars to any health system and some of the organisations that are helping to strengthen them.

While the humanitarian approach (explored further in Chapter 8) centres around the immediate delivery of health services, health systems strengthening supports sustainable public health systems. The next section focuses on two of the key pillars: health financing and the health workforce, both of which will be directly relevant to you in international health.

Health systems financing

Ways of financing healthcare systems vary from country to country. In most resource-rich countries, healthcare is financed through direct taxation or social insurance. Governments in many LMIC do not have the taxation revenue to meet the health needs of their populations. They are therefore financially dependent on donors and individual patients through user fees to make up the deficit (see Table 1.3).

User fees affect the decisions of individuals about whether and when to seek medical care. Those unable to pay for national medical care may opt instead for other healthcare providers like traditional healers or private practitioners. There is a burgeoning private healthcare industry in many LMIC, which is often unregulated.

Yet funding alone is not the only factor. Improved income distribution—even at low income levels—can accelerate improvements in health. Kerala, China, Cuba (see textbox below) and Sri Lanka are often cited as countries that have achieved high levels of health and education for their people before achieving high levels of income (Commission for Social Determinants of Health 2008).

Several LMIC countries have introduced a basic healthcare package which offers free services, especially for children and pregnant mothers, while other procedures incur nominal costs. A few LMIC now have health insurance programmes or community pre-payment schemes which are purchased by citizens. These schemes have had a massive impact on encouraging people to access healthcare.

Table 1.3 Comparison of health financing across five countries with similar populations

Country	Gross national income (£ billions) (2005)	Total expenditure on health as a percentage of gross domestic product (2006)	Individual expenditure on health as a percentage of total expenditure on health (2006)	External resources for health (i.e. aid) as a percentage of total expenditure on health (2006)	Per capita government expenditure on health at average exchange rate (£)
UK	2 263	8.2	12.7	0.0	2 908
Colombia	104	7.3	14.6	0.0	185
Democratic Republic of the Congo	6.9	6.8	81.3	51.9	2
Iran	187	6.8	49.3	0.1	109
Thailand	177	3.5	35.5	0.3	73

Source: World Bank 2006; WHO 2009

The Cuban health system: a personal perspective

....

"I have always been interested in history, the Spanish language and Latin America. When you add that to a medical career, Cuba seemed to me the ideal place to do a medical elective. I now know the Cuban health system from various perspectives. My wife and I have been patients in it, my children were born there, and I have studied there.

Cuba, although a Third World nation, boasts of life expectancy and infant mortality levels as good as developed nations. In Cuba, health-care is free to all and the country has one of the best doctor to patient ratios in the world. Its impressive record in public health is acknowledged by many including the Director-General of WHO, Margaret Chan.

The provision of health in Cuba is organised between family doctors, polyclinics offering minor outpatient services and hospitals offering specialist treatment and care. Healthcare is readily accessible even in remote areas. Cuba focuses heavily on preventative medicine. The uptake rate of vaccinations is high. Family doctors visit patients' homes with nurses and take a pro-active approach. Antenatal care is comprehensive. There are regular television, radio and billboard campaigns to promote awareness of health matters. The HIV rate is only 0.1 per 100,000, and HIV/AIDS specialist care is managed in one unit in the capital Havana. Cuba has even developed its own biotechnology industry which produces generic drugs and international health tourism, where patients travel from Europe and the United States to pay for services in Cuba, is a growing area.

Like all higher education courses in Cuba today, there are no tuition fees needed to study medicine. Upon qualification, the Cuban doctor must commit to a 5-year return of service to the Cuban government. This can include service overseas and long periods of separation from family and loved ones. Cuba regularly sends thousands of its medical staff to assist

➲

nations in Latin America, Africa and Asia, as well as training many doctors from LMIC at low cost. However, doctors can struggle to make ends meet on their wages, which are around $35 per month compared to the average of $20.

Sometimes there can be a lack of supplies in hospitals and pharmacies. It is not uncommon for family members to wash and change the bed sheets and bring meals to their relatives in hospital. There is concern about corruption in the system in that those who give doctors a 'gift' may get seen sooner or get a higher standard of care. There is also the worry that the brightest and most gifted doctors are sent abroad, thus denying Cuban citizens access to their skills. For instance, Cuba sends thousands of doctors and nurses to Venezuela in a deal for discounted oil. The counter argument is that this allows the government to spend more on its own health system rather than oil and its doctors gain experience which they bring back to Cuba.

Other nations look to Cuba as a possible model of what can be achieved with a limited budget. Health indicators such as life expectancy and infant mortality are as good as the United States. Whether you believe it is a good one to follow or not I shall leave to you. The system is by no means perfect but which one is?"

Captain (Dr) Stephen Hitchin, Senior House Officer in Infectious Diseases & Tropical Medicine, Royal Army Medical Corps

Aid

Governments in poor countries often rely on external aid to increase public spending on health. But there is not unanimous agreement that aid in itself is good and indeed there is significant criticism of its potential negative impacts. Arguments include absolving government and local communities from taking responsibility; and the tying of aid to donors' priorities rather than locally identified needs, thus weakening the system.

Aid comes in many forms and can be classified in several ways. It can be bilateral (from one government to another); multilateral (from pooled funds such as the European Union (EU) budget to another government); charitable donations; or a loan (e.g. World Bank, Asian Development Bank).

Funding may be paid directly to the local government or through intermediaries such as NGOs. It may go into the government's overall budget, support a single sector [sector-wide approach (SWAp)] or be in the form of technical assistance (intended to build capacity locally).

Governments and multilateral organisations are not the only ones supporting health. Private philanthropic groups such as the Gates and Clinton Foundations are increasing the total funding available. In some cases they support their own initiatives, and in others they act as health financiers, with other organisations managing funds on their behalf. The Global Fund for AIDS, TB and Malaria, which had a budget of just under $200 million in 2008, received 95% of its funding from donor governments.

Public Private Partnerships (PPPs), especially with pharmaceutical companies, are also proliferating with recognition that private corporations in partnership with NGOs and governments can be an effective way of improving healthcare in particular areas.

In recent years there has been increasing engagement between poorer LMIC and countries such as China, India and Brazil who were once regarded as part of the developing world but now are considered emerging economies. In Africa and Latin America, the Chinese government and businesses are supporting the development of health infrastructure such as hospitals and clinics. In 2006, China committed to support the development of 30 hospitals in Africa (Third World Network). India has recently signed an agreement with 47 African countries to the Pan-African E-Network which supports tele-medicine and tele-education (Nondo 2010).

The Paris declaration on aid effectiveness

While aid can help, it can also create problems. Different donors have different priorities pulling governments in different directions. Coordination is important and is one reason why countries around the world agreed in 2005 to the Paris Declaration on Aid Effectiveness. This was a comprehensive attempt to change the way donors and LMIC do business together, with increased harmonisation, alignment and focus on results with monitorable objectives and indicators.

Human resources for health

"The only route to reaching the health MDGs is through the [health] worker; there are no shortcuts."

Chen L et al. 2004

Money alone cannot bring about change. A skilled workforce, good management and health information systems are also essential. While free healthcare for the poorest is a step in the right direction, the next challenge is the chronic global shortage of health workers.

It is estimated that an additional 4 million health workers are needed to address the current global health needs. In 2006, the WHO identified 57 countries as having a critical shortage of health workers; 36 of these countries are in Sub-Saharan Africa (WHO 2006). For example, Zambia has only one doctor per 14,000 people (compared to one doctor per 600 people in the UK). In absolute numbers, however, the greatest shortage of health workers is in South East Asia with rapidly increasing population sizes (WHO 2006). In contrast, countries like Cuba, the Philippines and Egypt produce a surplus of health professionals for export around the world. So why is the distribution so unequal (Figure 1.2)?

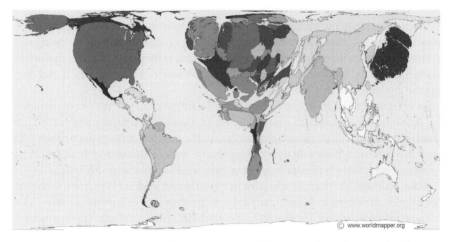

Figure 1.2 Distribution of nurses globally, 2004. (Territory size is based on the proportion of all nurses globally who work in that territory.) © Copyright SASI Group (University of Sheffield).

Emigration from poor countries to rich ones is not the only reason why those countries do not have enough health workers, although it certainly exacerbates the situation. Neither is it the migration within countries from public to private healthcare services, and rural to urban, though this also has an effect. The single most important reason why LMIC are hit hardest by the health worker shortage is because they have not trained enough of them (GHWA 2008). India trains only 10,000 nurses per year for a population of over 1 billion; Zambia trains 1,200 for 12 million. The UK meanwhile trains 25,000 for a population of over 60 million (Crisp 2010).

Where are all the health workers?

Movement or the 'brain drain' of health workers from poor to rich countries is often associated with the shortage of health workers in LMIC. In 2010 it was estimated that there were 224,005 registered doctors in the UK of whom about 25,767 were from India and 8,100 from Pakistan. Good for Britain but those figures represented respectively about 4% of India's doctors and 6% of Pakistan's. In Africa the problem is even more acute. It is estimated that Africa alone has lost 135,000 of her doctors and nurses to richer countries. The United Nations Conference on Trade and Development has estimated that each professional leaving Africa costs the continent $184,000 or $4 billion a year: one third of the official development funds to Africa (Marchal and Kegels 2003).

At the 63rd World Health Assembly in May 2010, the WHO Global Code of Practice on the International Recruitment of Health Personnel was adopted. The Code serves as an ethical framework to guide Member States in the retention and recruitment of health workers.

Since 2000 when the MDGs were agreed, LMIC have made pledges to address the issues of health workers. Most of them are working on designing, implementing and reviewing plans to increase and improve their health workforce. However, the lack of trained tutors and facilities, plus the lack of incentives to retain graduates, is challenging the implementation of these initiatives.

To counteract the shortage of health professionals, some LMIC have included lay workers in public health initiatives. For instance, Afghanistan and India have trained traditional birth attendants to increase the number of pregnant women who attended maternity clinics. In many countries the work of community health workers (paid and voluntary) is increasingly being integrated within the health system.

Many countries are training specialist cadres of health workers to perform tasks that are usually carried out by higher qualified professionals such as doctors or nurses. This is known as task-shifting. For example, in many LMIC, clinical officers (known by various names) are mid-level health workers that have much shorter training than a doctor but can perform some medical or surgical procedures (GHWA 2008). The qualification is often not recognised in Western countries, which can be limiting for the individual but can help their country avoid international 'brain drain'.

The history of medical training in Malawi

Formalised teaching of Western medicine in many LMIC did not start until the 1950s or later, so it is not surprising to find that they are less established and have a lower output than Western countries.

Take the case of Malawi, for example. Before Dr David Livingston's 1861 Zambezi expedition opened the door to Western medicine, only traditional doctors or herbalists existed. Even today many patients coming to the hospitals bear the scarification mark on their bodies, suggesting the Sing'anga (traditional herbalist) has been there first.

Blantyre mission hospital was built in 1896 and it became possible to teach local staff. However, training was limited by previous levels of education as until the 1940s there were no secondary schools in Nyasaland. In 1926 Nyasaland saw the return of its first local doctor, Dr Daniel Malekebu, who had studied medicine in Nashville, Tennessee. By the 1950s things were looking up, with a greatly increased health budget which made it possible to expand training. By 1961 'Medical and Laboratory Assistants and Midwives [were being] trained at Blantyre, Medical Aides at Lilongwe, Health Assistants and Assistant Nurses at Lilongwe'.

The Malawi Medical Association was formed in 1964—the same year as independence was achieved—and had a membership of 27 (including mission and private doctors). Their hope was that the 32 Malawian medical students training abroad (mainly in Britain, but also Uganda, India and South Africa) would return by 1969, but unfortunately this did not happen.

Extracts from *The Story of Medicine and Disease in Malawi* by Michael and Elspeth King.

The first and only medical school in Malawi was established in 1991. It has grown from an intake of 10–15 students per year and a handful of Malawian faculty members, to a programme with a medical student intake of 60–100 per year with 110 faculty members, of whom approximately 67% are Malawians. To date the college has graduated over 250 medical doctors (http://www.medcol.mw/).

A short term response to this health worker crisis is the recruitment of medical personnel from outside their countries. In the medium term, LMIC are building capacity within their health sectors with the help of development partners, focusing on training and motivating local health workers. In the long run, there is a renewed global call to transform global health education to produce health systems and professionals that cater for the needs of the communities that they serve rather than their professional desires. These are all strategies that you can contribute to as a UK health professional working in international health.

The UK response

The UK has actively taken a lead in responding to global health issues. The government provides significant financial support both in bilateral aid and to global organisations such as WHO (its second largest donor after the United States). British organisations have pioneered health partnerships and many other global health initiatives. UK academic institutions have an extremely strong track record in global health research. Individual health professionals who combine international work with a UK career are becoming more visible. This last section reviews key developments in the UK response to global health.

What the government is doing

> "Britain's nurses, midwives and medical teams are some of the best in the world and can help to give low and middle-income countries the skills needed to improve women's health."
>
> *Andrew Mitchell, Secretary of State for International Development, June 2010*

In 2007 the then UK government produced two reports that addressed the UK's role in global health. The first, *Global Health Partnerships,* looked at how UK experience and expertise could be used to support health initiatives in LMIC and how this would be for our mutual benefit. It led to a range of initiatives including:

- a pension contribution scheme for UK health professionals working overseas (unfortunately now discontinued)
- the development of a new grants scheme for health partnerships run by THET and the British Council
- the International Health Links Centre, which is a repository of information on health partnerships (http://www.ihlc.com)
- the creation of a £20 million fund over 4 years to support health partnerships and volunteering managed by THET and the consultancy firm HLSP.

The second report, *Health Is Global*, had a wider remit. It promoted a multisectoral approach, differing from international health which traditionally focused exclusively on healthcare systems. It argued that the eradication of global poverty and disease would, in turn, protect the health of the UK population.

Later the same year, the UK government launched the International Health Partnership (IHP), a global initiative, to coordinate the funding commitments of donors around a single national health plan. The IHP is being administered by WHO and the World Bank and has evolved to become the Global Health Partnership and Related Initiatives (IHP+) in recognition that its launch coincided with a range of other initiatives with similar goals.

The UK's Department for International Development (DFID) funds governments bilaterally and stations health advisors in many supported countries. These advisors provide advice on policy and planning as well as overseeing UK support to health budgets, increasingly through SWAps. The 2009 DFID white paper *Eliminating World* DFID's health priorities include the acceleration of the health-related MDGs, humanitarian assistance, the strengthening of health systems and public health initiatives.

In 2010, the UK's Department of Health (DH) released the *Framework for NHS Involvement in International Development*. This has been developed to provide greater clarity on how NHS agencies and individuals can best maximise their potential to contribute in a sustainable and appropriate way to capacity building in LMIC. The framework covers five areas including the UK policy context, principles of effective engagement, benefits to the NHS of international work, architecture for NHS activity in LMIC and finally good practice for organisations, individuals and employers (see more in Chapter 13).

What British organisations and individuals are doing

British organisations and individuals are incredibly active in international health.

> "We can play our part in improving health globally while developing leadership and other skills in the NHS and further building and sustaining our international networks."
>
> Sir David Nicholson, KCB CBE, NHS Chief Executive (England)

There are many students and health professionals who give up their time to support projects, campaign on global health issues, and volunteer overseas.

NGOs like THET have supported institutional health partnerships between the UK and health organisations in LMIC for over two decades. There are over one hundred of such partnerships across the UK. Voluntary Service Overseas (VSO), Médecins sans Frontières (MSF), Doctors of the World, Merlin and other volunteer organisations recruit UK health professionals for overseas placements to support the implementation of health plans in LMIC. Other charities such as Oxfam are campaigning for free basic healthcare for all and raising awareness of the negative consequences of unregulated private health practitioners.

Through their international departments, professional associations and the Royal Colleges support exchanges and training opportunities for health professionals overseas. Health professionals from Diaspora groups or LMIC backgrounds have also set up their own organisations or support projects in their originating countries.

What you could do

The time has never been better to join these endeavours to improve global health. The professional colleges and associations are increasingly supporting international work, and health partnerships have received more funding. There are more training posts with opportunities to work abroad, and efforts to formalise global health training and qualifications. Finally, global health courses are proliferating and there is increased global health content in undergraduate curricula.

This chapter has given you a whistle-stop tour of some of the biggest themes in global health. The impact of these issues on work overseas is explored in later chapters. If you are intrigued, read on to find out whether international work is for you.

REFERENCES

Broadhead RL, Muula AS (2002). Creating a medical school for Malawi: problems and achievements. *British Medical Journal* 325(7360):384–7.

Centers for Disease Control and Prevention (2009). Global measles mortality, 2000–2008. *Morbidity and Mortality Weekly Report* 58(47):1321–6.

Chen L, Evans T, Anand S, Boufford J, Brown H, Chowdhury M, Cueto M, Dare L, Dussault G, Elzinga G (2004). Human resources for health: overcoming the crisis. *Lancet* 364(9449):1984–90.

Clemens MA, Petterson G (2008). New data on health professionals abroad. *Human Resources for Health* 6:1–10.

Commission on the Social Determinants of Health (2008). *Closing the Gap in a Generation: Health Equity Through Action on the Social Determinants of Health.* Geneva, World Health Organization.

Crisp N (2010). *Turning the World Upside Down: The Search for Global Health in the 21st Century.* London: Royal Society of Medicine Press.

Dowden R (2008). *Africa: Altered States, Ordinary Miracles.* London: Portobello Books.

Global Forum for Health Research (2011). http://www.globalforumhealth.org/ (accessed 31 January 2011).

Global Health Watch (2005). *Global Health Watch 2005–2006: An Alternative World Health Report*. London: Zed Books.

Hicks J, Allen G (1999). *A Century of Change: Trends in UK Statistics Since 1900* (Research paper 99/111). London: House of Commons Library.

Joint Learning Initiative (2004). *Human Resources for Health: Overcoming the Crisis*. Cambridge (MA): Harvard University Press.

King M, King E (2007). *The Story of Medicine and Disease in Malawi*, 4th edition. Self-published.

Levine R (2007). *Case Studies in Global Health: Millions Saved*. Centre for Global Development. Sudbury, MA: Jones & Bartlett Publishers.

Marchal B, Kegels G (2003). Health workforce imbalances in times of globalization: brain drain or professional mobility? *International Journal of Health Planning and Management* 18(Supplement 1):89–101.

McColl K (2008). Europe told to deliver more aid for health. *Lancet* 371(9630): 2072–3.

Nondo B (2010). *India Launches Pan African E-Network. AllAfrica.com.* 26 August 2010. http://allafrica.com/stories/201008270647.html (accessed 31 January 2011).

Organisation for Economic Co-operation and Development (2009). *Measuring Aid to Health. OECD-DAC, 27 November 2009.* http://www.oecd.org/dataoecd/44/35/44070071.pdf (accessed 31 January 2011).

Pillars of the Health System. *Disease Control Priorities Project.* http://www.dcp2.org/pubs/PIH/7/ (accessed 31 January 2011).

Rowson M (2007). *Health systems - why they need to be at the heart of all our societies*. BMA International Department. Chapter 1 in Improving health for the world's poor: what can health professionals do?

Task Force for Scaling Up Education and Training for Health Workers, Global Health Workforce Alliance (2008). *Scaling Up, Saving Lives*. Geneva: Global Health Workforce Alliance.

Third World Network (2006). *China: Doubles Aid and Investment to Africa.* http://www.twnside.org.sg/title2/finance/twninfofinance010.htm (accessed 31 January 2011).

UNAIDS (2010). *Report on the Global AIDS Epidemic*: 2010 Geneva: UNAIDS.

UN Inter-Agency Group for Child Mortality Estimation (2010). *Levels and Trends in Child Mortality. Report 2010.* New York: United Nations Children's Fund.

United Nations (2010). *The Millennium Development Goals Report 2010*. New York: United Nations.

World Health Organization (2006). *World Health Report: Working Together for Health*. Geneva: World Health Organization.

World Health Organization, UNICEF, UNFPA and The World Bank (2010). *Trends in maternal mortality: 1990 to 2008*. Geneva: World Health Organization.

World Health Organization (2009). *World Health Statistics Report 2009*. Geneva: World Health Organization.

World Health Organization. (2011). *Q&A: Health Systems*. http://www.who.int/topics/health_systems/qa/en/index.html (accessed 31 January 2011).

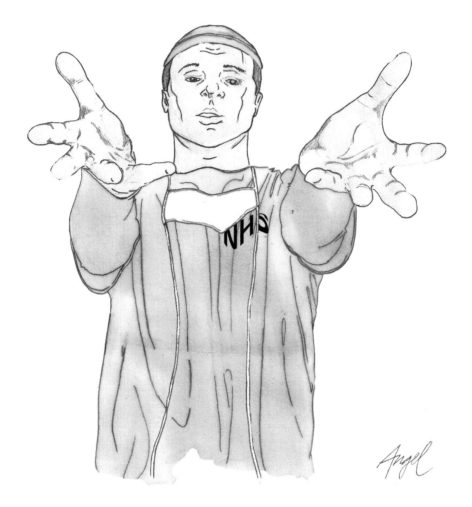

Angel

CHAPTER 2

Why do it?

The previous chapter will have left you in no doubt that there is still plenty of work to be done in international health. Health workers who use their skills to help overseas are becoming more common and more visible. But why should *you* get involved?

International work is not for everyone. Working in a different country and culture is very appealing to some and not at all to others. As aid worker Matthew Bolton puts it, "one has to have pretty strong (and perhaps strange) motivations to want to leave one's home, family, and friends and go live in war zones and situations of poverty".

Author Helen Fielding described four types of aid workers in her satirical book *Cause Celeb*: the missionary, the mercenary, the misfit and the broken-hearted. Indeed, it is said that some interviewers for international health jobs ask applicants "What are you running away from?" In reality, people choose to work in international health for a whole range of personal and professional reasons. Sometimes these reasons can hinder your work overseas. In this chapter, we describe some of the most common reasons to work in international health. Think about which best captures your motivations and how you could avoid the potential pitfalls.

Common motivations for international work

1 For moral reasons
2 For religious reasons
3 For the love of travel
4 For the adventure
5 For the lifestyle
6 To help your homeland
7 For professional and personal development

For moral reasons

> "I wanted to help balance out the distribution of doctors in the world."
>
> *Neurologist, Rwanda*

The international demand for experienced healthcare workers is high and the statistics are often shocking, as seen in Chapter 1. With these glaring inequalities in access to trained health workers, you may feel a moral obligation to work in areas of greater need.

> "In the UK I was seeing about 10 patients a day, giving them specialist one to one consultation. Here in Bangladesh, I can see up to 70 or more patients in a day. I feel I am making much more of a difference, making much better use of my skills."
>
> *Consultant, Bangladesh*

But bear in mind . . .

Many people often talk about 'doing good' and 'making a difference'. It is best to leave all notions of 'saving the world' behind. You will quickly realise that while you may be able to make a difference to some individual lives (much as you would in your own country), your overall impact is likely to be small in the grand scheme of things. This can be frustrating, and you may become disheartened. However, there are many ways in which you can maximise the impact of your time overseas: see Chapter 13.

For religious reasons

> "I went to Malawi because as a Christian I wanted to serve those who had been neglected by others. I think every Christian should be concerned about the poor."
>
> *Palliative care doctor, Malawi*

> "I got involved in humanitarian health work for moral reasons, because I believe that it is part of my obligation as a doctor and as a Muslim. It also gives me personal and professional fulfilment."
>
> *Emergency physician, worldwide*

Faith can be a very strong motivating factor for working overseas. Many religions speak of the need to help those less fortunate than you. Providing health by sharing your skills can be a way to answer this call. Feeling spiritually fulfilled can help to counter any career and financial worries from your time abroad. Also it can be very refreshing to be in cultures that are less secular than the UK.

> "At university, I feel the odd one out to have a strong faith. Whereas here in Africa, it's the norm. I have had many great conversations with people about their faith, which I would rarely have at home."
>
> *Medical student on elective, Kenya*

Faith-based organisations (FBOs) provide a proportion of health services in many LMIC. For example, over 40% of the health services in Malawi are delivered by CHAM, the Christian Health Association of Malawi. In these establishments, religious worship often forms a part of daily working life.

> "I enjoy being able to merge my professional life with my religious beliefs. Part of our working day includes hospital staff and family members coming to pray by the patient's bed."
>
> *Nurse, South Africa*

But bear in mind . . .

If you are going overseas for religious reasons, be sensitive to the local context. In many places, religion is a source of ethnic tension and violence, so be careful not to add to this. If you want to evangelise, it is usually better practice to keep this separate from work (although in FBOs, the distinctions can be blurred). If you go with an organisation, some will have a policy of neutrality or non-religiosity. As an ambassador of that organisation, you should be willing to conform to these policies abroad.

For the love of travel

If you love travelling, then international health offers the chance to experience a new culture and people from a far closer perspective than a holiday can allow. As a health professional, you will gain insight into cultural beliefs and the wider influences in health beyond the biomedical perspective. Living and working in a new place is one of the best ways to become more open-minded, lateral thinking and better at your job once you return.

"My visits to South Africa have given me a much richer understanding of my patients' perspective. Now when I see African patients in my clinic, I understand that these patients are coming from a country where antiretrovirals are rare and everyone has lost several family members to AIDS. So when I give them their diagnosis, and then reassure them that there's treatment available and it's a chronic disease now rather than a death sentence, of course they don't believe me. I now reinforce this over several clinic visits, and I can see the fear gradually going away."

Paediatric HIV nurse, South Africa

But bear in mind . . .

Language can be a barrier, and learning some of the local dialect is always worth the effort (see Chapters 6 and 9). Cultural nuances can be difficult to grasp, and you can still be an outsider after many years in one place. Jobs in international work can be extremely busy and if you have planned lots of local travel, you are likely to be disappointed. Do try to schedule some respite breaks early in a nice location so you can look forward to these during tough times at work.

For the adventure

"My favourite experience was training female Community Health Workers in Afghanistan. I had to travel to very remote mountainous areas by donkey to persuade the elders to let them be trained."

Nurse and midwife, Afghanistan

For adventure seekers, there are many exciting opportunities out there and it can be tempting to choose your destination on the basis of maximum adventure. Fast-paced environments such as emergency relief can seem particularly attractive.

But bear in mind . . .

Often, excitement goes hand in hand with risk to security and personal wellbeing.

"Security incidents constantly threaten the projects. We are in contact with war lords and community leaders, especially when running the mobile clinics. I had a friend who was killed."

Nurse, MSF

Remember that the destinations that look the most adventurous from afar are usually those with very disrupted health systems and infrastructure, making humanitarian or development work much harder and potentially less rewarding than work in more stable places. In conflict zones, the local situation may be so unstable that travel may be limited by your organisation or peacekeeping forces. You may end up never leaving the safety of your compound and workplace, and in reality have much less adventure than your peers in more stable countries. Consider your options carefully: see Chapters 5 and 11.

For the lifestyle

> "I travel by banka (small fishing boats) and have hibiscus and orchids outside my window."
>
> *Nurse and midwife, Philippines*

When you work overseas, you could be living in a tropical paradise where you are the only foreigner for miles around, or a cosmopolitan capital city with much better quality of life than in the UK. Even if your salary is less than it was in the UK, your income is likely to buy you a more comfortable lifestyle with bigger accommodation, domestic staff or frequent travel. And if you are a volunteer or receiving a basic stipend, better weather and beautiful surroundings can make time overseas seem idyllic compared to the UK.

> "People think we are saints, sacrificing our life to work 'in Africa'. But we have a much nicer and more comfortable life here than we did back home. There are nice restaurants, good schools for our children, and lots of cultural events happening. Good weather for most of the year. I work in a private hospital so we have many of the resources we need. At home we have four domestic staff working at the house: a cook, cleaner, nanny and guard. This is standard here, even for the locals. You can live a very nice life here if you want, with weekends by the beach, or visiting national parks. Yes, we are on lower salaries, but life is cheaper here. It will be very hard to go back. I think we might try Asia next."
>
> *Doctor, Kenya*

But bear in mind . . .

Although having such a lifestyle is hugely enjoyable and provides local employment and revenue, try to keep an eye on your primary purpose. The vast majority of the population will never be able to enjoy such a lifestyle. Be careful not to distance yourself or create barriers between the very people you are here to help. If you employ local staff, try to set an example with fair pay and safe working conditions.

To help your homeland

The UK is home to a large Diaspora population. If you are part of this, you may want to use your skills to contribute to health improvement in the region of the world you come from. Having a foot in both worlds may help you to bridge the cultural gap and allow you to work more effectively. Language skills in particular will be of great advantage.

> "My parents come from Pakistan and I often visit and have close ties there. I volunteered to go back after the 2005 earthquake as I felt it was something I had to do. After all, I have been so lucky to be born and educated in Britain and now that I am a doctor I feel a huge sense of responsibility about giving something back—here in the UK but also in Pakistan. I really appreciate how privileged a position this is and every time I go back I find more reasons to return. The need is huge, resources are extremely limited and the people are so grateful for whatever you can do for them. For me, going back to help is a no brainer."
>
> *GP, Pakistan*

But bear in mind . . .

Recognise that you may face some problems on your re-entry to your homeland. If you are a first-generation emigrant, you may face resentment or distrust from those who remained behind. If you are second or third generation, you may find yourself in a halfway house of understanding some cultural references but missing many others. Some compatriots are likely to view you as a foreigner or outsider, despite your origins. Also be aware that a large proportion of the malaria cases seen in the UK every year are due to Diaspora not taking malaria prophylaxis during visits home.

For professional and personal development

> "My time on elective made me much more confident in my clinical skills. I came back knowing I could pick up diagnoses even in a different health system and language. It also confirmed to me that I wanted a career working overseas, and I have focused my training around this goal."
>
> *Junior doctor, on elective in Madagascar*

Whatever your role overseas, you will undoubtedly grow professionally and personally. You are likely to be given greater responsibility and opportunities that stretch you much further than back at home. The next chapter goes into more detail about the potential benefits of your time abroad.

> "I was not finding my work or life in England entirely rewarding. I wanted to develop personally and professionally and thought that Tanzania could give this to me. And it was a definite step up as here I have a range of roles: supervision, teaching and working in forensics. I am also working with drug and alcohol users, which is something I had never done before."
>
> *Clinical psychologist, Tanzania*

But bear in mind . . .

Be aware of your limitations. Any healthcare is not always better than dangerous healthcare. For example, if you are a student on elective, you should always work under supervision and not take on responsibilities beyond your capability. But if you are a bit more senior, you might find you are the most experienced person around. And this can mean that your professional development is limited in the long term due to lack of guidance. Personal development will also stall if you are exhausted and mentally drained. Although the need can be overwhelming, try to avoid taking on more than you can cope with—burnout is a real possibility.

Conclusion

Health workers go overseas for many reasons. Think about your real motivations for going abroad and try to balance these to ensure they don't detract from the overall goal of improving local health.

Whatever your reasons, you will be playing a role in the wider context of knowledge transfer and health improvement. Some of this will benefit you but burden the NHS. Some will benefit the NHS, but weaken other health systems. Some will contribute to international health but leave you considerably disadvantaged. The following chapter looks at the rewards and challenges of international work from an individual, organisational and global perspective.

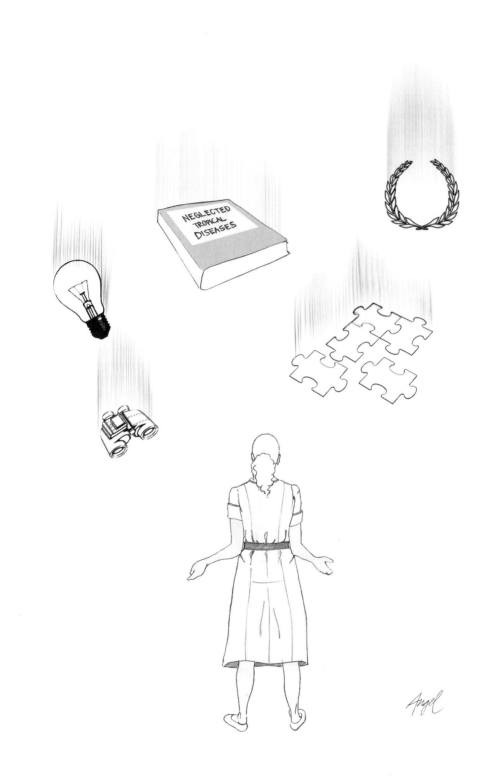

CHAPTER 3

The rewards and challenges

The overwhelming majority of people who have worked overseas say that it has enriched their lives. But overseas work is not all adventure and excitement. It's important to be aware of the potential difficulties in order to manage your expectations.

This chapter explores both the rewards and challenges of international health work from three perspectives: you, your host and the bigger picture (including the NHS) (Figure 3.1). Its aim is to give you a very honest view of international health work today. Chapters 12 and 13 then go on to explore how you can maximise the rewards and minimise the challenges during your time overseas.

Despite encountering some or all of these challenges, most people come away inspired and fulfilled—and ready for more.

For you

Rewards

Setting up a cholera hospital, travelling to remote health clinics, coordinating vaccination campaigns in war-torn countries—it's easy to see why the change from the daily grind of NHS service is one of the major rewards of international work.

> "You're doing what you thought you would when you dreamed of being a doctor."
>
> *Emergency doctor, Guyana*

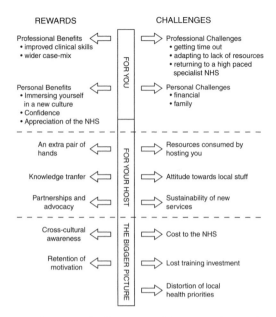

REWARDS   CHALLENGES

FOR YOU

Professional Benefits
- improved clinical skills
- wider case-mix

Professional Challenges
- getting time out
- adapting to lack of resources
- returning to a high paced specialist NHS

Personal Benefits
- Immersing yourself in a new culture
- Confidence
- Appreciation of the NHS

Personal Challenges
- financial
- family

FOR YOUR HOST

An extra pair of hands

Resources consumed by hosting you

Knowledge tranfer

Attitude towards local stuff

Partnerships and advocacy

Sustainability of new services

THE BIGGER PICTURE

Cross-cultural awareness

Cost to the NHS

Retention of motivation

Lost training investment

Distortion of local health priorities

Figure 3.1 Rewards and challenges of international health work.

With so many health workers returning to international work time and time again, it's clear that they must be getting something out of it for themselves. Here we describe some of the main benefits, both professional and personal.

PROFESSIONAL BENEFITS

The professional benefits of working overseas are usually framed within the narrow scope of clinical training, such as improved diagnostic skills and a wider case-mix. Whilst these are undoubtedly benefits of international work, they are surprisingly not the most commonly cited by health workers returning home.

Benefits of international work cited by VSO health workers

- Being forced to challenge the status quo, and learning how to do this effectively
- Working across the entire range of their skills, rather than a narrow specialism
- Getting involved in service issues that would be dealt with by managers in the UK
- Learning to take a wider, population-based approach to healthcare needs and priorities
- Learning to understand the needs and issues of multicultural communities in the UK
- Having to learn practical (non-clinical) skills such as budget and project management

➲

- Gaining confidence and the ability to question decisions, assumptions and attitudes of colleagues
- Delivering good patient care with limited resources, and overcoming severe resource limitations
- Learning to spot examples of waste and an appreciation of how to improve efficiency in the NHS

Compiled by Baringo Consulting, for VSO

Many of these skills are management functions, which can be difficult to get experience of whilst junior. However, these are skills that are looked highly upon when applying for more senior or consultant posts (Figure 3.2). Indeed, staff who can demonstrate their ability to stretch limited resources and increase efficiency will be highly valued in the NHS in coming years. Chapter 14 offers advice on how to frame or 'sell' competencies achieved overseas when you return home.

"The benefits of overseas work in an NHS career are often best understood by doctors and others with managerial responsibilities."

Banatvala and Macklow-Smith (2007)

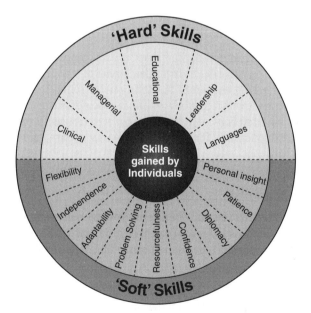

Figure 3.2 Skills gained by an individual health worker during his or her international placement. Reproduced with kind permission of Tribal Newchurch (2010) adaptation of Lord Darzi's Next Stage Review (2009).

Advanced presentations and exposure to unusual pathology will enhance your clinical learning. Clinical skills that may have stagnated in the UK become honed in an environment where ordering a CT scan is a luxury. Confidence in diagnostic skills and selectivity in investigations is usually associated with increasing seniority in the NHS, and will be looked upon favourably if demonstrated at a more junior level.

> "Many doctors have never seen a patient with full-blown AIDS before they come here. It's a real education for them."
>
> *Malawian junior doctor, teaching hospital, Malawi*
>
> "I feel more confident in my clinical judgement since coming back from South Africa. I know that with limited resources I managed to look after some of the sickest patients I have ever had to treat. I now try to order fewer tests to confirm my diagnosis, and I'm much more conscious of what they cost."
>
> *Surgical trainee, South Africa*

Finally, the increased responsibility which is frequently shouldered overseas can develop a true sense of clinical leadership. You may spot many areas where you have the knowledge to improve quality of care, which needs to be coupled with the sensitivity to bring local staff along with you. Innovation can be difficult to implement in the NHS, but your successes in a less rigid environment may give you the confidence to push through change back at home.

> "The royal colleges and their faculties are in general agreement that doctors and nurses can benefit from being part of a well-structured overseas programme, be it research, development, or relief. There are at least five areas where overseas work enhances professional development: empathy, accelerated clinical learning, a cost conscious approach to health care, taking responsibility for developing quality of care, and flexibility."
>
> *Banatvala and Macklow-Smith (2007)*

PERSONAL BENEFITS

If you have only travelled overseas, working in a country will give you a very different experience. Immersing yourself in a culture is very different to just travelling through it. You are likely to gain a much deeper understanding of its people and may develop a lifelong relationship with your host country.

> "I have a real affection for Madagascar after my time working there. I felt much more enveloped into people's lives and formed much deeper friendships than other countries I have just visited on holiday."
>
> *Junior doctor, Madagascar*

International work gives you a greatly increased confidence, both in yourself and your clinical abilities. The knowledge that you can be inventive and adaptive if the situation requires remains with you after your return and frequently enhances your work in the now seemingly stable NHS. Returning workers also cite a greater understanding of global issues, a wider world-view and a clarification of personal priorities. Comparisons with other health systems can also produce a renewed and healthy appreciation of the NHS. Finally, living in LMIC can leave you with a deep gratitude of your own situation and life security.

Challenges

There are undoubtedly many personal challenges to working overseas. For a start, you are faced with the logistical problems of getting time out of the system, minimising the impact on your personal finances, and maintaining your close relationships whilst away.

> "It took me 6 months to arrange out of programme time for research (OOPR) with my deanery. They weren't obstructive, but each form seemed to need signing in triplicate by the powers at be. I'm glad I started soon after I got my grant, otherwise my departure could have been delayed."
>
> *Medical researcher, Malawi*

Whilst you're there, you will have to adapt to a lack of resources, different practices and values, and high rates of mortality and morbidity, all perhaps whilst speaking a different language.

If you have been overseas for a while, coming back to the UK and to a high-pace and very specialist NHS can be difficult. You may have to find a new job or get your time away recognised. You are likely to meet resistance and scepticism regarding the benefits of international work, whatever your stage.

> "After my return, my financial difficulties were really because of the problems finding work and settling back into working life in England on my return. I hadn't been able to (nor had I wanted to) keep my previous job, and it was nigh on impossible to apply for jobs whilst I was still in Tanzania. This meant the first 3 months of being back in England I was furiously job-hunting, and having to live off my savings at that point. A bit of bad luck that there was a general election and very few services were advertising in April/May of that year!"
>
> *Psychologist, Tanzania*

Despite this, many health professionals have successfully combined international work with an NHS career. In Chapters 4 and 15, we describe the career pathways of several people who have achieved this seemingly impossible task. All these personal challenges are examined in more detail in later chapters.

For your host

Rewards

AN EXTRA PAIR OF HANDS

Chapter 1 described the health worker shortage faced by many LMIC. If you've ever been on-call for the third day in a row, with 10 cases waiting, and one of your team phones in sick, then you will recognise the utter relief of having an extra pair of hands appear. Simply being another member of an under-resourced and struggling team can make the world of difference in weakened health systems.

Even more appreciated are extra members of the team with specialist skills. Specialist training requires qualified trainers, and is therefore in its infancy in many LMIC. Those with niche skills can make a big impact, especially if clinical work is combined with training local workers. For example, Dr Vicky Lavy set up a paediatric palliative care service in Malawi, where she lived and worked for 10 years. She designed a 5-day introductory course in palliative care, which was subsequently developed into a national training programme.

> "When I arrived at the hospital, the paediatric ward was overflowing with children dying from AIDS. My palliative care service focused on both symptom control and getting these children out of hospital. There was also a sister adult palliative care service doing similar work. The nurses found this type of care very empowering and asked for more training. 1,585 people have now taken the training course—6% of all health workers in the country—and there are 25 palliative care teams around the country."
>
> *Dr. Vicky Lavy, Malawi*

KNOWLEDGE TRANSFER

For local clinicians working in resource-poor environments, continuing professional development is often very limited. Visiting clinicians have a valuable role to play in keeping local colleagues up to date with the latest evidence and guidance.

> "They discuss lots of rare conditions when diagnosing a child. Although these are unlikely, it is really interesting to listen to these conversations— we learn so much through them. It is very enlightening."
>
> *Malawian junior doctor, paediatric research unit, Malawi*

The contrast can also highlight the good practice and strong systems in your own workplace. Those training sessions or checklists that have been tedious up to now may suddenly seem to have a point.

"After a really awful resuscitation attempt in a 25-year-old man which was unsuccessful, I could really see why protocols on resuscitation are helpful. The emergency trolley hadn't been refilled, there was no face mask by the patient's bedside, and no-one was leading the team. A local doctor and I made up a protocol after this, and ran a couple of practice scenarios. The next resuscitation was much smoother."

Emergency doctor, Guyana

But it's not just a one-way transfer of knowledge from the NHS to LMIC. Many health workers encounter different ways of doing things overseas, which they feel would add value back in the NHS. There are many things that the UK has learned from poorer countries. Innovative models such as conditional cash transfers for lifestyle changes, nurse-led clinics for chronic diseases and polyclinics were all established overseas, before being trialled in the UK.

"I spent 3 years as a GP in a rural health centre in Brazil. These centres provide comprehensive primary care for a geographical population of about 5,000 people. There was a strong focus on health education and motivational interviewing to improve lifestyle choices. I was very impressed with the ethos and the effects of this approach. In fact, I am now starting some research looking at what the NHS can learn from this model."

GP, Brazil

PARTNERSHIPS AND ADVOCACY

"I took 6 months out and went to work in a large referral hospital which had one qualified occupational therapist. He was very motivated but had very little support. He was so appreciative of me being there, working together and sharing ideas. It really gave him a boost to have extra support and we continue to stay in contact and share ideas now I am back in the UK."

Occupational therapist, Uganda

You can act as a gateway for the development of partnerships and networks with health institutions across the world. You might help establish a Health Link (see page 66) with a UK organisation and help recruit other volunteers in areas of need. A motivated, committed health professional with an awareness of local issues advocating on their behalf in a resource-rich environment can be of great benefit for your host.

> "I am still involved with the organisation I worked with for 9 months in Tanzania. I am involved in a research project with local colleagues and I am also helping them develop projects to continue some of the work that I started."
>
> *Psychologist, Tanzania*

Challenges

RESOURCES CONSUMED BY HOSTING YOU

Do not underestimate the burden put on your hosts. The administrative time, induction and supervision (if necessary) by senior clinicians are all resources that could have been spent on patients or local staff. If you are on a long-term placement, this will eventually pay off. But if you are only there for a short time, you may leave just as you are finding your feet.

Compare it to starting a new job in the NHS. It usually takes at least a month until you are familiar with the particular ways of your new ward or consultant. It might take even longer for you to feel that you are really on top of the job and its requirements. Now think about doing this in a completely different health system, with a different case-mix and perhaps in a different language. When do you feel you would be contributing to the system, rather than draining it?

> "Continuity of longer-term support provided by experienced UK staff was most valued by southern partners. Multiplicity of short-term inputs (e.g. two week visits) were—with the exception of specifically-requested technical areas—poorly regarded."
>
> *James et al. (2009)*

This is particularly true for electives, where students do not usually contribute substantially to patient care (see Elective Advice below).

> ### Elective advice
> ....
> "Providing elective opportunities for medical students . . . imposes a significant administrative burden on the host country. Given that their resources are already limited, sometimes severely, students should make every effort to avoid imposing unnecessary burdens on their hosts. Students should also think carefully about the levels of supervision that can realistically be provided by senior colleagues in resource-poor settings. It is important to recognise that the primary obligation of health professionals is to their patients. Educationally, the priority will also be the training and development of health professionals who are working within the country."
>
> *British Medical Association (BMA) (2009)*

ATTITUDE TOWARDS LOCAL STAFF

> "Malawians are very polite and friendly. They are used to working together. However, they do not respond well to being ordered around. Lots of new doctors come here, and start ordering juniors and nurses around. People start thinking, 'Don't come all this way just to dictate to me'."
>
> *Malawian junior doctor, teaching hospital, Malawi*

However great your appeal as an extra member of the team, this will not excuse arrogance or rudeness towards the local staff. It is very easy to disregard the clinical expertise and contextual wisdom of your new colleagues in the midst of your glorious arrival from the supposedly knowledge-rich UK. It is even easier to act in the same way you do at home and inadvertently offend your colleagues through cultural misunderstandings. The ways of getting things done in the pressure cooker of Western work environments can be far less effective overseas. Feel your way cautiously at first, until you know what is acceptable, and view your colleagues as a source of knowledge. You have as much to learn from them as they have from you. Chapters 10 and 11 explore these issues further.

> "It's best to view your experience as an exchange of knowledge, rather than one-sided. We have much local knowledge and well-honed clinical skills, which are very valuable."
>
> *Malawian junior doctor, teaching hospital, Malawi*

SUSTAINABILITY OF NEW SERVICES

> "A previous set of doctors set up computerised forms for us to enter in data about HIV-positive children. However, when they left, there was no-one with the skills to look after the equipment. So it just sits in a corner now."
>
> *Malawian junior doctor, paediatric research unit, Malawi*

When you arrive in a new placement, the possible improvements that could be made may be striking. However, hold yourself back. Health institutions in LMIC are littered with unused equipment and failed innovations that well-meaning foreigners have tried to put into place without assessing the local situation. Valuable staff time can be diverted into implementing these innovations, even when they are almost certain to fail.

Ask yourself whether there are practical reasons why the current system is in place? Who has the skills to maintain the new equipment? Who will run the service after you leave? Chapter 13 gives advice on how to make sustainable improvements.

For the bigger picture

> "The ultimate beneficiaries from UK professional health workers gaining international experience are NHS patients in the UK."
>
> *Liam Donaldson, Chief Medical Officer for England (1998–2010)*

It can be difficult to convince those who have not been involved in international health that the NHS will be improved as a result of your work. But all the hard and soft skills mentioned above will be put to good use in an NHS that is increasingly focused on value for money and wise resource allocation. Clinicians with management skills will be needed to lead on new initiatives to provide high quality care and increased productivity under tough economic conditions.

Benefits

CROSS-CULTURAL AWARENESS

> "It's not until you've visited a country where 1 in 4 people have HIV; where there is a coffin shop at the entrance to the hospital; where most of the children in your clinic are orphans; that you truly understand the fear of your African patients in the UK."
>
> *Paediatric HIV nurse, South Africa*

The NHS serves a diverse population: 7.9% of the UK population today is non-white, and an estimated 590,000 people arrived to live in the UK in 2008 (Office for National Statistics 2001 & 2008). These populations often have different disease burdens to the general population and different attitudes towards disease and healthcare. For example, nearly 40% of new HIV diagnoses in the UK in 2008 were among black Africans, of whom the majority had acquired their infection abroad (Health Protection Agency 2008).

Your international work can give you a deeper understanding of your patients' culture, including health beliefs, social constraints and ways of dealing with illness. This will allow you to provide more effective care for them, particularly in terms of communication and health education. Indeed, targeted Health Links in countries from which your immigrant populations originate can provide excellent opportunities to improve care for these groups.

Many immigrants come to the UK with little English and no understanding of how the health system runs, which can lead to poorer quality of care as a result. Increased awareness of different cultural norms can lessen your frustration when those new to the country do not fall in with the standard way of doing things.

"I had to sit down with my African patients and explain the NHS appointment system. It was difficult for them coming from a culture where there are no set appointments. I could fit them in if they turned up 2 hours late, but the doctor—well, that was another matter."

Paediatric HIV nurse, Luton

RETENTION AND MOTIVATION

". . . Of great benefit to the staff and patients within the NHS, doctors return to the UK reinvigorated and refreshed, bringing both new ideas and new energy to their careers and feeling that they have made a significant contribution to the global health community."

BMA International Department (2009)

Many health workers return from their time overseas revitalised and full of renewed enthusiasm for their work. Combining international work with a career in the UK can make you more motivated and appreciative of the NHS.

"Each time I get back from my trips, I get a boost of enthusiasm for my day-to-day work. Morale is very low in the NHS at the moment. Seeing the situation for health workers in Sierra Leone makes me grateful for what I have."

Consultant surgeon, Sierra Leone

Using your skills to help people who have so much less and for whom your intervention makes such a difference can be extremely rewarding. Motivated, satisfied staff are likely to provide better quality care to their UK patients and remain in the NHS.

To think about

The NHS needs to makes savings of £20 billion in the next few years, and staff cuts have been proposed. However, the cost of replacing a member of staff can be between 50% and 150% of their annual salary (including recruiting and training a replacement, and associated loss of productivity).

Could the NHS retain valuable personnel and make savings by allowing more breaks in staff contracts to work overseas? Could staff members facing reduced hours accumulate these and spend the extra time overseas?

Challenges

COSTS TO THE NHS

In the short term, the NHS will often lose out through your time away (especially on longer trips). This may be through:

- Salary costs for your replacement
- Increased burden on your colleagues if no replacement is found
- Loss of your expertise, which may lead to decreased quality of care

These are very tangible losses, which are likely to be felt keenly by your line managers and colleagues. However, it is easy to lose sight of the war when you're fighting battles every day. International work will benefit you, patients and the NHS in the long term. Be prepared to justify your time away by citing some of the benefits above.

LOST TRAINING INVESTMENT

Training health professionals is expensive. It is estimated that a doctor in the UK costs on average £250,000 to train to qualification (Chitty and Cooke 2004). However, it is assumed that these training costs will be reimbursed by the service provided to the NHS. Given that skilled health professionals are such valuable commodities, should the NHS allow its investment to be frittered away on work overseas? Worse still, these expensive professionals may never return to the NHS and instead work full-time in international health.

On the other hand, some would argue that the NHS has a responsibility towards the global health community. Before immigration rules changed in 2007, health workers from outside the European Economic Area were specifically recruited for the NHS. The culture of outmigration developed by this policy in LMIC still has enormous ramifications today. Moreover, it greatly reduced training costs for the NHS. It is estimated that the UK has saved some £65 million in training costs between 1998 and 2002 by recruiting Ghanaian doctors, whilst Ghana has lost £35 million of its training investment to the UK (Martineau *et al.* 2004). Furthermore, the majority of UK health workers do return to the NHS after a period overseas, with skills and training that benefit the NHS.

> "Almost all of MERLIN's volunteer doctors have returned to the NHS: a far cry from the popular myth that doctors interested in working overseas are trained by the NHS, only to be lost to developing countries for ever. In fact most return after 1 or 2 years overseas and are a valuable resource to trusts or health authorities."
>
> *Banatvala and Macklow-Smith (2007)*

DISTORTION OF LOCAL HEALTH PRIORITIES

Chapter 1 described the different types of aid available, and its delivery through vertical (disease-specific) or horizontal (sector-wide) programmes. Although the tide is slowly turning, much overseas funding is still designated to key diseases such as HIV/AIDS and malaria. This approach has led to great advancements in their management, for example the roll-out of antiretroviral drugs. However, in weakened health systems, it can lead to the sidelining of patients with 'ordinary' diseases (such as diabetes or neglected tropical diseases) and the deprioritisation of less novel but highly effective interventions such as improved nutrition and vaccination.

"The doctors will stop in front of each child's bed and look through the notes to see whether they have HIV. If the child is positive, they spend a long time with him or her, and sort out all their medical problems. If the child is negative, they move onto the next one: they are no longer interested. In a funny way, it is a blessing to have HIV in this ward."

Malawian junior doctor, paediatric research unit, Malawi

Most health workers engaged in international work are not involved in such strategic decisions. However, you will be representing your organisation and as such need to agree with its approach. Consider whether your organisation responds to local needs or imposes its own objectives. Will your work strengthen the local health system or will it distort priorities?

"Our funding was from PEPFAR [The United States President's Emergency Plan for AIDS Relief] and we focused exclusively on HIV/AIDS. We would pay per diems for local staff to attend our training workshops, but this would often be the equivalent to a month's wage for some. This took them away from their patients in the district general hospital. We built an expensive new day centre for HIV-positive patients. Even for general medical complaints the HIV-positive patients ended up avoiding the less-resourced district general hospital in favour of the day centre, completely distorting care pathways and clinical care."

General Practitioner (GP), Mozambique

To think about

Imagine if an Ethiopian NGO descended on Camden Town in order to sort out the homeless population. They would not have a nuanced understanding of the risk factors for this population like psychiatric illness or past military service. They would not understand our complex social care system. They would probably distribute *injera* bread thinking this is what they would want in the same situation. How would the homeless population respond—grateful, resentful or confused? Do we make the same assumptions when we set up NGOs overseas?

Conclusion

This chapter has offered an insight into the numerous rewards of international work, and also the diverse challenges. The idea of international work is extremely appealing, but the reality can be much harder. Remember that, on balance, most people would say that it's worth it. Be aware of the potential difficulties, and keep your expectations in check. The next chapter will allow you to assess whether the time is right for you to engage in international work.

REFERENCES

Banatvala N, Macklow-Smith A (2007). Integrating overseas work with an NHS career. *British Medical Journal* 314(2):7093.

British Medical Association (2009). *Ethics and Medical Electives in Resource-Poor Countries—A Toolkit.* London: BMA.

British Medical Association International Department (2009). *Broadening Your Horizons: A Guide to Taking Time Out to Work and Train in Developing Countries.* London: BMA.

Cooke L, Chitty A (2004). *Why Do Doctors Leave the Profession?* London: British Medical Association (Health Policy and Economic Research Unit).

Health Protection Agency (2008). *HIV in the United Kingdom: 2008 Report.* London: Health Protection Agency.

James J, Minett C, Ollier L (2009). *Evaluation of Links Between North and South Healthcare Organisations.* London: DFID Health Resource Centre.

Martineau T, Decker K, Bundred P (2004). 'Brain drain' of health professionals: from rhetoric to responsible action. *Health Policy* 70:1–10.

Office for National Statistics (2001). *Census 2001.* Newport: ONS.

Office for National Statistics (2008). *Migration Statistics 2008 Annual Report.* Newport: ONS.

Royal College of Nursing (1996). *The Benefits of Overseas Experience.* London: RCN.

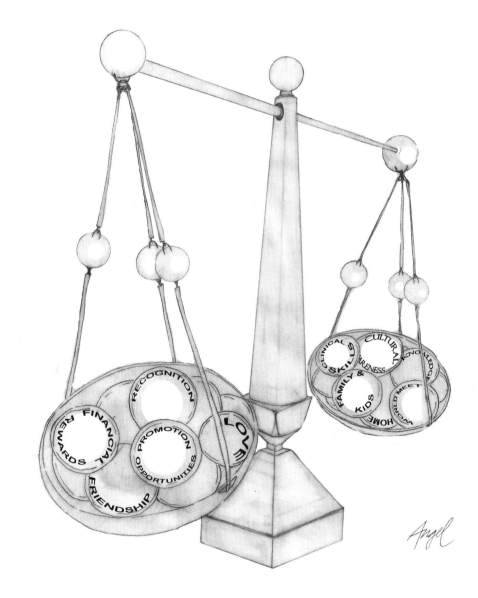

CHAPTER 4

Is it possible?

International work is a treasured goal of many health professionals. But there are lots of reasons why going overseas may not feel possible for you right now. You may be in the middle of your undergraduate or postgraduate training. You may have just had a baby or bought a new house. You may be wondering how you can possibly find the time to go away whilst fitting in all your clinical, managerial and personal responsibilities.

When interviewing the many health professionals who contributed to this book, the same stumbling blocks to international work came up time and time again.

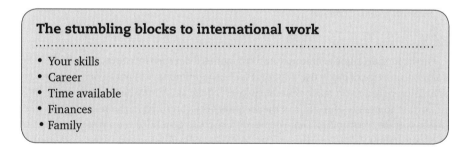

The stumbling blocks to international work

- Your skills
- Career
- Time available
- Finances
- Family

This chapter describes the opportunities for international work within each of these restrictions. Having weighed up these personal and professional considerations, you can then move onto looking at specific placements in the next section. Remember that many people have made international work a reality despite these barriers. To motivate you, we have included throughout the chapter the careers trajectories of health professionals who have successfully combined a UK career with international work. It was possible for them—it could be possible for you too.

You may come out of this exercise with the realisation that now is not the time to go overseas. Don't worry—at the end of the chapter we highlight some alternative ways to spend your time until the right moment comes along.

Your skills

The most important consideration before you embark on international work is what you have to offer. What skills do you have? Are you confident in them? Will you give more to your host country than you take?

Overseas work can be extremely challenging in terms of workload, lack of supervision and case variety. You need to be confident in your clinical and personal ability to handle situations that even senior professionals might find demanding. You may decide that it is better to gain these skills in the UK, in a well-supervised environment that promotes learning, and go overseas at a later date (excluding electives). Indeed, most recruiting organisations will not accept those with less than 2 years' professional experience. If you've committed to international work but are below this threshold, see the last section for things you can do to prepare yourself in the meantime.

> "When the earthquake hit Haiti, I desperately wanted to go out there and help. But as the news reports came through I realised that I just didn't have the skills they needed. In that environment there is little supervision so being able to perform the necessary operations independently is essential. It was hard to admit that I wasn't going to be that useful, but I did not want to be put in a situation where I knew patients had sub-standard care because I didn't have the correct skill set."
>
> *Surgical trainee, London*

On the flipside, some people may be too qualified for certain locations. A cardiothoracic surgeon won't be of much use if there is no cardiopulmonary bypass available—unless s/he is prepared to do more general surgery. Niche skills may be in demand, but it is important to match your skills to the location very carefully. In the majority of placements you are likely to find that you need to be more generalist than you are used to in the UK. Chapter 7 gives more details on recruiting organisations and assessing whether you are right for the job.

While being an English speaker is a great advantage, additional languages, such as French, Spanish or Arabic, are highly valued by recruiting organisations and may enhance your chances of recruitment and choice of location. For many consultant assignments, a working knowledge of the appropriate language(s) is often an imperative. Chapter 6 looks into this issue in more detail.

Career

The ideal time to go on a placement overseas is when you really want to. However, it is most easily arranged during a natural pause in your career, e.g. in between jobs, at the end of a training rotation or after retirement. Although looking for new jobs and being accessible for interviews may curtail your ideal placement, it is an unforgettable way to use up those extra months and hopefully enhance your CV.

For the majority who are not lucky enough to be at this point, fitting international work around an upwards career trajectory is challenging. Options for taking time out include:

• **Annual or study leave**

   This is the best option for short-term placements. If you're doing work for an institutional partnership (see below), see if your employer will allow you to use study leave rather than your holiday allowance. Study leave can also be granted for longer periods.

• **Sabbatical**

   These are usually only for senior professionals or academics and you would have to demonstrate that the placement has considerable educational or research benefits. Your salary may or may not be paid during this time—check your local policy.

• **Unpaid leave of absence**

   This is usually for placements of less than 3 months and has the same terms as a career break.

• **Career break**

   A career break is an extended period of unpaid leave available for approved purposes and subject to specific conditions. All NHS employers are now required to have a policy on career breaks, so you shouldn't need to resign to work overseas, but you will need to meet certain conditions (see Box 4.1).

- **Time out of programme (OOP)**

  This option is only for those doctors in a post-graduate training programme and is described in more detail below.

Box 4.1: NHS career breaks

- Breaks can be between 3 months and 5 years (taken as a single period or several breaks), although more than 2 years is rarely granted.
- You will need to have at least 12 months' NHS service.
- The agreed length of the break will depend on your length of continuous service and the needs of the service.
- You would not be allowed to take up paid employment with another employer during the break, but international organisations are usually exempt.
- If the break is for less than a year, you should be able to return to your old job, if practical.
- For breaks of more than a year, you should be able to return to a similar job.
- If you take an agreed career break, your NHS employment is treated as continuous and you should be able to return at an equivalent salary level, however you may lose out on salary increments due during this time.
- Other benefits dependent on your length of service (such as pension benefits) will be suspended for the duration of the break.
- You should stay in touch with your employers during the break and arrange refresher training on your return as necessary.

For more information, contact your human resources (HR) department.

As individual professions have different training requirements and career paths, we highlight some of the relevant issues by profession below.

Doctors

(See Figures 4.1 and 4.2)

- **Medical students**

  Most medical students can undertake an elective period of clinical work in another country in their fourth or fifth year. This is usually for 2–3 months and up to 40% of medical students go overseas during this period (Miranda et al. 2005). Make the most of your elective, as it can be the first chance you have to see if international work is genuinely for you. Start thinking about where you want to go early and begin planning at least a year ahead. Chapter 7 has more advice.

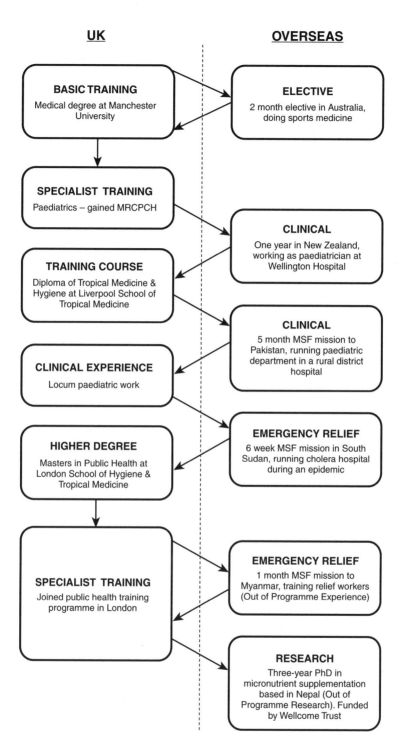

UK

OVERSEAS

BASIC TRAINING
Medical degree at Manchester University

ELECTIVE
2 month elective in Australia, doing sports medicine

SPECIALIST TRAINING
Paediatrics – gained MRCPCH

CLINICAL
One year in New Zealand, working as paediatrician at Wellington Hospital

TRAINING COURSE
Diploma of Tropical Medicine & Hygiene at Liverpool School of Tropical Medicine

CLINICAL
5 month MSF mission to Pakistan, running paediatric department in a rural district hospital

CLINICAL EXPERIENCE
Locum paediatric work

EMERGENCY RELIEF
6 week MSF mission in South Sudan, running cholera hospital during an epidemic

HIGHER DEGREE
Masters in Public Health at London School of Hygiene & Tropical Medicine

SPECIALIST TRAINING
Joined public health training programme in London

EMERGENCY RELIEF
1 month MSF mission to Myanmar, training relief workers (Out of Programme Experience)

RESEARCH
Three-year PhD in micronutrient supplementation based in Nepal (Out of Programme Research). Funded by Wellcome Trust

Figure 4.1 Career diagram of specialist registrar in public health, Delan Devakumar.

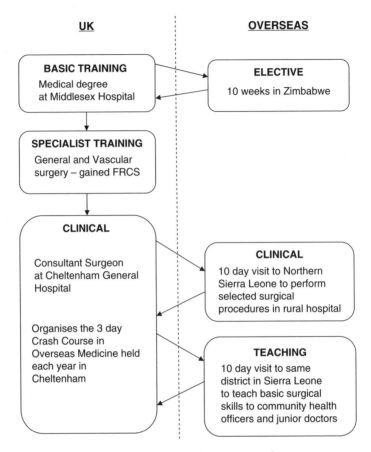

UK

BASIC TRAINING
Medical degree
at Middlesex Hospital

ELECTIVE
10 weeks in Zimbabwe

SPECIALIST TRAINING
General and Vascular
surgery – gained FRCS

CLINICAL

Consultant Surgeon
at Cheltenham General
Hospital

Organises the 3 day
Crash Course in
Overseas Medicine held
each year in
Cheltenham

OVERSEAS

CLINICAL
10 day visit to Northern
Sierra Leone to perform
selected surgical
procedures in rural hospital

TEACHING
10 day visit to same
district in Sierra Leone
to teach basic surgical
skills to community health
officers and junior doctors

Figure 4.2 Career diagram of consultant vascular surgeon, Mark Whyman.

- **Training grades**

   Clinical skills gained through international work can be useful for many specialities, particularly infectious diseases, paediatrics, obstetrics, trauma and orthopaedics, and public health. Good times to go overseas are either between Foundation Year 2 and starting core/speciality training, between core and speciality training if this is applicable for your intended speciality, or once you are on a speciality training scheme. The considerable advantage of the latter is that you can return to a guaranteed training post and retain your National Training Number.

   If you do go away during your training scheme, you will take time out of programme (OOP). A maximum of 3 years can be taken OOP, but this is not usually granted during the final year of training (see Box 4.2).

   Some OOP periods can count towards the award of your Certificate of Completion of Specialist Training (CCST). Weigh up whether you feel you will gain specialist

Box 4.2: What is time out of programme?

Trainees may take a period of time out of their speciality training programme for one of a number of reasons:

1 For approved clinical training in a post that already has prospective approval from the GMC (out of programme training—OOPT)
2 For clinical experience in a post that will not count as training time and towards a CCST (out of programme experience—OOPE)
3 For research (out of programme research—OOPR)
4 For a career break (out of programme career—OOPC). This is different to maternity or adoption leave, which does not count as time out of programme.

competencies overseas and can cut down on your remaining training time, versus the extra time spent in training back here. You can generally count up to two years of OOPR time towards your CCST. However, some curricula don't allow this, so check with your training college.

For OOPT, you will have to make an application for prospective GMC approval through your deanery. It all depends on whether adequate training supervision is available at the host location. If you are awarded OOPT, you will receive your basic salary (i.e. without on-call supplements) during your placement. It will also definitely count towards your CCST. Full details of OOP guidance can be found in of *The Gold Guide* and the BMA has also published excellence guidance.

A few fortunate trainees are on training schemes that include the option of an overseas post. The most established is probably the VSO/RCPCH fellowship (see Box 4.3). The general practice 3-year vocational training scheme was previously felt to be too short to allow trainees to go away during it. However, an increasing number of 4-year schemes are being offered by deaneries, with a 12-month OOPE offered between the second and third year. Severn Deanery is leading the way: see http://primarycare. severndeanery.org/recruitment.

Find out more

- *The Gold Guide: A Reference Guide for Postgraduate Specialty Training in the UK*. Medical Specialty Training (England), 2010. *http://www.mmc.nhs. uk/specialty_training_2010/gold_guide.aspx*
- *Broadening your Horizons: A Guide to Taking Time Out to Work and Train in Developing Countries*. BMA International Department, March 2009. *http:// www.bma.org.uk/international/working_abroad/broadeningyourhorizons.jsp*
- See Appendix 2 for specialty-specific resources.

- **Consultants and retirees**

  Consultants are very much in demand, especially to support training. However, they will usually have to take a sabbatical or come to a special agreement with their employers for medium- or long-term placements. Some consultants use their annual leave to do training, service work and/or teaching. These trips can be extremely busy, particularly surgical service visits where a high number of operations are performed, and you may come away feeling like you need a holiday to recover.

Box 4.3: VSO/RCPCH fellowship

This fellowship is essentially a 1-year OOPE, working with VSO overseas. Fellows have previously worked in Malawi, the Gambia, Cambodia, Indonesia, Kenya, Uganda, Tanzania and Namibia.

Structured support is available from the College, including an in-country mentor and a College mentor in the UK, who you will liaise with remotely. VSO provides a living allowance, accommodation, health insurance, return flights, pre-departure and in-country training, along with GMC registration and indemnity insurance costs. As it's an OOPE, you won't receive your UK salary but may be paid a local salary.

Specialist trainees from ST3 onwards are eligible, and feedback from previous Fellows is that the best time to go is post-MRCPCH, with 1–2 years' middle-grade experience.

In fact, the most convenient time for many doctors to go overseas may be in early retirement. You are likely to be missing clinical work, you haven't yet developed that golf obsession and you are still in good health. Your clinical expertise will be in great demand for both service work and training, and you may wish to consider a medium- or long-term placement. However, be aware that some organisations do have an upper age limit or they abide by the partner country retirement age.

Find out more

- *Advice for Retired Members on Volunteering and Global Health*. British Medical Association, July 2010. *http://www.bma.org.uk/international/working_abroad*
- *Re-tyred not Retired: Healthcare Mission in Later Life*. Christian Medical Fellowship, 2008. Order Reference: Ret0805. This booklet recounts the stories of 11 retired doctors who shared their skills overseas.

Nurses and midwives

(See Figure 4.3)

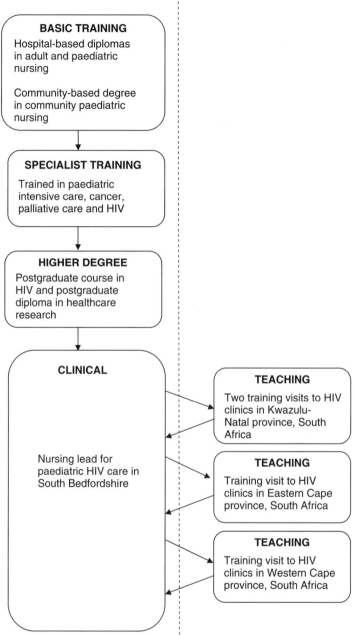

Figure 4.3 Career diagram of paediatric HIV nurse, Marielle Connan.

- **Students**

  Nursing and midwifery electives are now widely available. They are usually taken in year 2 or 3. Although it is still not as common to go overseas as for medical students, more nursing students are taking this opportunity to experience other health systems and different ways of practicing. Consider applying for the WHO Nursing Internship scheme (see below).

WHO nursing internships

The WHO Nursing and Midwifery Office is offering opportunities for nursing students to be involved in global health policies and systems through its internship programme.

Internships are for 8 weeks and these are open to degree students who are finishing their programme from an accredited school. There is also an off-site programme for interns requiring in-country work with a WHO Collaborating Centre lasting at least 8 weeks. Each participant will work with a faculty adviser at a WHO Collaborating Centre who will provide on-site guidance and supervision.

More information is available at *http://www.who.int/hrh/nursing_midwifery/ internships/en/*.

If an elective is not available, it is possible under current rules to take a year out and return later to your studies. Indeed, if you are undertaking a full-time 3-year programme, you do have 5 years (including any breaks for illness, etc.) in which to complete the course. However, think about whether your contribution would be greater after qualification and a couple of years' experience.

Find out more

- *Overseas Electives for Nursing Students*. Royal College of Nursing, 2008. Available for members at *http://www.rcn.org.uk/*
- *For Student Midwives Undertaking Overseas Elective Experience: Frequently Asked Questions*. Royal College of Midwives, 2005. *http://www.rcm.org.uk/college/students/*
- *Preparing for your Nursing or Midwifery Elective Overseas*. Christian Medical Fellowship, 2004. *http://www.cmf.org.uk/internationalministries/electives. asp*. Written from a Christian perspective.

- **Qualified nurses**

  Under current rules any activity undertaken overseas (including practice and CPD) can count towards the requirements for maintaining registration. The International Humanitarian Community at the RCN may provide useful support.

It is a network of RCN members who have worked or are currently working in global health. It aims to share experiences and to raise the profile of international humanitarian work. See http://www.rcn.org.uk/development/communities/specialisms/international_humanitarian.

Find out more

....

- *Working with Humanitarian Organisations: A Guide for Nurses, Midwives and Healthcare Professionals* (2nd edition). Royal College of Nursing, 2010. Publication code 003 156. *http://www.rcn.org.uk/*
- *General Information on Working Abroad.* Royal College of Nursing, 2008. *http://www.rcn.org.uk/*
- *Guidelines for Members Experiencing Problems Whilst Working Overseas.* Royal College of Nursing, 2008. *http://www.rcn.org.uk/*
- *Midwives Working Overseas.* Royal College of Nursing, 2008. Available for members at *http://www.rcn.org.uk/*
- *Thinking About Working Abroad?* Royal College of Midwives, 2006. *http://www.rcm.org.uk/college/international*

Allied health professionals

(See Figures 4.4 and 4.5)

- **Students**

  Electives for students on allied health training courses are not well established, but it can be done in summer holidays. However, expect to do much of the leg work yourself and anticipate some bureaucracy. Approach your course organiser as a first step.

"I arranged a 2-month elective in India during the holidays between my third and final clinical years. This wasn't usual at all, and I was the only one in my course who did it. I told my tutor that I was going to do it, but otherwise had to organise it all myself. I had just done a big clinical block, so felt confident in my abilities. In order to publicise my experiences, I made a video documentary for the student branch of the British Pharmaceutical Association, which was on their website for ages."

Pharmacist, India

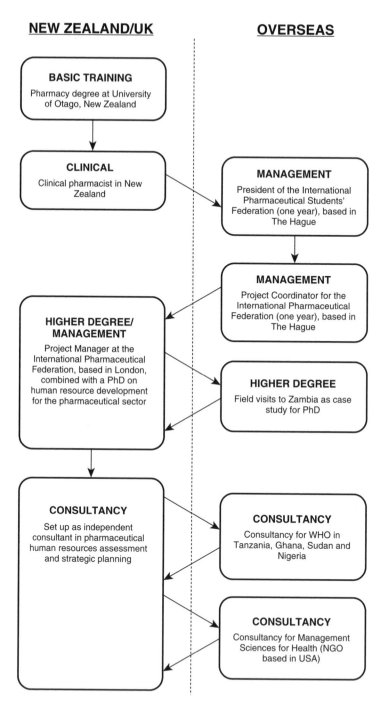

NEW ZEALAND/UK　　　　　　**OVERSEAS**

BASIC TRAINING
Pharmacy degree at University of Otago, New Zealand

CLINICAL
Clinical pharmacist in New Zealand

MANAGEMENT
President of the International Pharmaceutical Students' Federation (one year), based in The Hague

MANAGEMENT
Project Coordinator for the International Pharmaceutical Federation (one year), based in The Hague

HIGHER DEGREE/ MANAGEMENT
Project Manager at the International Pharmaceutical Federation, based in London, combined with a PhD on human resource development for the pharmaceutical sector

HIGHER DEGREE
Field visits to Zambia as case study for PhD

CONSULTANCY
Set up as independent consultant in pharmaceutical human resources assessment and strategic planning

CONSULTANCY
Consultancy for WHO in Tanzania, Ghana, Sudan and Nigeria

CONSULTANCY
Consultancy for Management Sciences for Health (NGO based in USA)

Figure 4.4 Career diagram of international health consultant and pharmacist, Tana Wuliji.

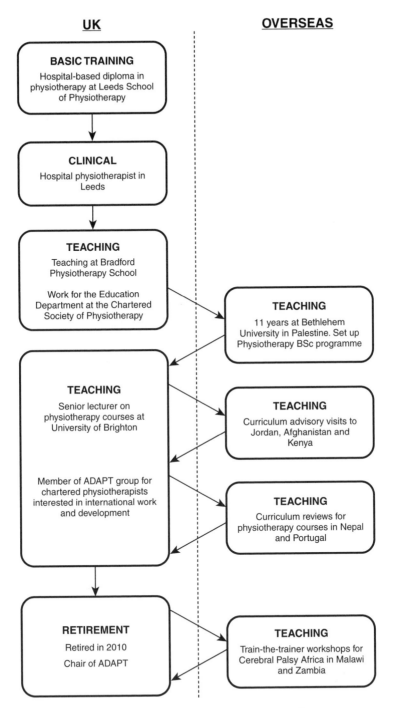

UK

OVERSEAS

BASIC TRAINING

Hospital-based diploma in physiotherapy at Leeds School of Physiotherapy

CLINICAL

Hospital physiotherapist in Leeds

TEACHING

Teaching at Bradford Physiotherapy School

Work for the Education Department at the Chartered Society of Physiotherapy

TEACHING

11 years at Bethlehem University in Palestine. Set up Physiotherapy BSc programme

TEACHING

Senior lecturer on physiotherapy courses at University of Brighton

Member of ADAPT group for chartered physiotherapists interested in international work and development

TEACHING

Curriculum advisory visits to Jordan, Afghanistan and Kenya

TEACHING

Curriculum reviews for physiotherapy courses in Nepal and Portugal

RETIREMENT

Retired in 2010

Chair of ADAPT

TEACHING

Train-the-trainer workshops for Cerebral Palsy Africa in Malawi and Zambia

Figure 4.5 Career diagram of physiotherapist, Lesley Dawson.

Find out more

- *Arranging an Overseas Radiography Placement/Elective*. Imaging in LMIC Special Interest Group of the Society and College of Radiographers. *http://www.idcsig.org/page6.html*
- *FAQs on Working Overseas*. Royal College of Speech and Language Therapists, email: information@rcslt.org
- *Volunteer Advice Pack*. Communication Therapy International, 2008. *http://www.commtherapyint.com*
- *International Orthoptic Association Guidance for Orthoptists Considering Work in LMIC*. Rowena McNamara, 2010. British and Irish Orthoptic Society, email: bios@orthoptics.org.uk

Relevant allied health organisations

ADAPT

This is a specialist interest group for chartered physiotherapists working in international health and development. They provide useful information on overseas work and contacts, and organise an annual study day. Recent research on their members showed that most placements were in paediatrics, neurology and teaching, and the most common condition treated was cerebral palsy. *http://www.adapt-physio.org.uk*

Communication Therapy International

This was set up by a group of UK speech and language therapists with overseas experience in 1990. It aims to serve as a network for all those interested in working in communication disabilities overseas, not just qualified specialists. Their advice pack offers lots of useful tips for working in a different culture and resource-poor setting, and how to make your work sustainable. *http://www.commtherapyint.com*

Imaging in LMIC Special Interest Group

This group of the Society and College of Radiographers is a network of professionals working in the field of medical imaging looking to share knowledge and best practice for the advancement of radiography in LMIC. They have produced advice based on their experiences and hold regular study days. *http://www.idcsig.org*

International working group of the British Association of Occupational Therapists

This group progresses international business on behalf of the Association. For more information contact the lead officer for international activity. *http://www.baot.org.uk*

Qualified

Many allied health professionals spend time working overseas and your professional association may be able to put you in touch with other members who have worked abroad. See also the special interest groups opposite. CPD will be your own responsibility, and you will need to demonstrate a portfolio of all your CPD activities to maintain registration with the Health Professions Council (see Chapter 12).

Managers

Many hospitals in low-income countries cite management issues as one of their main hurdles. Specific hospital management training is rare, with clinical staff usually covering management tasks as part of their job. The shortage of management expertise is a significant barrier to strengthening many health systems. Unfortunately, it is not as common for non-clinical hospital managers in high-income countries to take time out to work in LMIC compared to clinicians. However, their skills are equally needed.

Hospital managers wishing to work overseas will encounter a range of opportunities, from taking on full-time management jobs to project planning and implementation. The 2-year NHS graduate management training programme used to have a component where an overseas placement was possible, but unfortunately this is no longer the case. Some hospital managers are also involved in their institution's Health Link, where they provide advice and mentorship to fellow managers overseas. More senior managers may find consultancy appropriate for them (see Chapter 5).

Find out more
....

- Conn C, Green C (2006). *Effective District Health Services in Low and Middle-Income Countries: A Busy Manager's Guide to the Literature*. IDS. This book will give you a flavour of management overseas and help you identify other publications on the different topics that you might have to deal with as a district manager.

Other non-clinical staff

Other support staff often find that their organisational skills and inside knowledge of health organisations make them attractive to humanitarian organisations in non-clinical roles. These include logisticians, communications, human resources and finance roles. See Chapter 7 for an overview of the kind of people needed by ten major organisations.

Time available

If you have a full-time job in the UK, engaging in international work will inevitably involve taking time out. How much time can you offer? Two weeks of annual leave? A 3-month sabbatical? Or would you consider a career break of a year or two?

We have divided international work up into three broad categories: short (<1 month), medium (1–6 months) and long-term (>6 months) placements. These definitions will be used throughout the book. Below, we describe the common types of work undertaken in each time frame.

Short-term placements

> **Common types of short-term work**
>
> ....
>
> • Emergency relief
> • Visits to undertake elective surgery
> • Health Link visits (see box below)
> • Teaching and examining
> • Consultancy

Those involved in short-term visits will often need to be experienced in their field and have a very specific remit with clear deliverables for their visit. It's good to understand how the visit fits in to a wider strategy, how it has been planned and how it will be evaluated. This type of placement is well suited to people working within the NHS or universities who want to share their expertise overseas when time allows. As this type of work is the most attractive, it will also be the most competitive.

Examples of short-term placements include emergency work, teaching, examining or visits with a specific purpose, e.g. carrying out a needs assessment. It is unusual for one-off clinical placements to be less than a month unless they are part of a planned programme, e.g. cataract operations.

The first response to an emergency may require short-term placements, but by its very nature this work is unpredictable and therefore difficult to plan in advance. Junior health workers may have to fit this work into annual leave. More senior professionals may be able to come to an understanding with their institution if they regularly go on relief missions and are able to arrange suitable cover for their duties (see Figures 4.2 and 4.3).

> **Health Links: Hospital and university twinning programmes**
>
> ....
>
> These organisational partnerships are growing in popularity in the UK and are supported by the Department of Health and DFID. The essence of Links is that
>
> ➲

they are long-term partnerships which respond to the demands of the overseas partner. The UK organisation (e.g. a hospital) draws from its own staff base to find individuals who are able to respond to these priorities, and often focuses on capacity building. Reciprocal visits from overseas staff back to the UK are also a key feature of many Links.

A Health Link allows the individuals involved to contribute towards long-term, mutually agreed objectives through short-term visits. However, the individuals who take part in the exchange visits will be determined by the technical expertise required by the overseas partner institution. If your experience does not fit into this, there will always be opportunities to support the planning and strategy development for the Link and learn more about your partner institution.

The International Health Links Manual, 2009 has details about what a Link is and how to set up and maintain a long-term institutional partnership. See *http://www.thet.org.uk*.

Medium-term placements

Common types of medium-term work

- Electives
- Clinical practice
- Rehabilitation/Development
- Research
- Consultancy

A placement of 1–6 months can seem the ideal compromise between a whistle-stop few weeks and the logistical challenges of longer periods. For those new to international work, it can give you a feel of what it is like living and working abroad without the long-term commitment. It is also an ideal introduction to tropical diseases and working in a different health system and can be incorporated into time off at the end of training rotations or between jobs (see Figure 4.1).

If you are a junior doctor and planning a medium- or long-term placement, see if you can use your taster week(s) during foundation training or study leave to prepare for your trip. You could visit your destination to meet your local contacts or go on relevant courses.Alternatively, undertaking a research project with an international aspect could give you a first chance to live and work abroad. For example, many Masters degrees offer a research project overseas. For longer projects, you will probably be linked to a local university or research institute (see Figures 4.1 and 4.4). The Medical Research Council has research centres in the Gambia and Uganda which regularly host UK trainees and professionals. See Chapter 11 for some of the specific challenges of doing research in resource-poor environments.

Long-term placements

Common types of long-term work

....

- Clinical practice
- Teaching
- Rehabilitation/Development
- Research

Longer-term placements can be the most attractive of all posts. When you are new to a country it takes time to adjust, understand the local culture and make a lasting impact, and this usually requires a period of more than a few months. The memories, experiences and friendships forged through a long-term placement are often what people are seeking from international work and there is certainly no better way to get to know a country.

These types of placements are most valued by overseas institutions as you will have enough time to really settle in and make a difference to them. But as these types of placements require the most commitment on your behalf, international agencies often have difficulty recruiting for these types of posts. So if you are prepared to commit a year or more to work overseas, the range of placements available with the right skills will be significant.

While short-term, topic-specific teaching visits can be valuable, a placement of 6 months or a year allows you to take responsibility for a specific area of curriculum, freeing up other teaching staff. You will be able to get to know the institution and students, and contribute to the next generation of health workers in that country (see Figure 4.5). Formal teaching experience such as this is often looked upon favourably by postgraduate deaneries, and can be an excellent addition to your CV. Teaching duties can also be supplemented with clinical experience at the local teaching hospital in order to keep your skills fresh.

See Chapter 5 for more detail on all these types of work.

Money

International work is rewarding in many ways, but few of these involve money. View your time overseas as one rich in new experiences, new friends and new horizons—but not as a way to get rich. Well-paid overseas posts are usually only available to those with considerable international experience or niche skills who work for international organisations as consultants. In addition to lower or no salary, you may have to pay your pension or National Insurance contributions. Practicalities such as insurance, flights and freight costs can eat into your savings.

In reality, you are likely to lose out financially as a result of an international placement. This is certainly not a reason to forego the opportunity, but don't be under any illusions and consider your financial situation carefully before making arrangements.

"When I said I was going to do 6 months' unpaid work in South Africa, most people thought this was financial and career suicide. At the time I was so in debt, it didn't really matter. My advice to anyone else is that you have to be aware that you will pay for your time abroad and miss out on your NHS salary. Now several years later, I'm still paying off loans while my friends are buying smart cars. It helps to know that the experience was worth it. I would do it all again—a hundred times over."

Surgical trainee, South Africa

Salary

Whether you receive a salary or not is very much dependent on what you do. Possibilities range from well-off to pauper (see Box 4.4). Chapter 7 goes into more detail about the costs covered by major organisations.

Box 4.4: The range of salaries available in international work

💰💰💰 Consultancies and specialist assignments offer competitive salaries and benefits.

💰💰 If you are on secondment from your organisation, or on OOPT or OOPR as a medical trainee, then you will be receiving roughly your UK salary. Some organisations also pay a UK salary equivalent on longer-term placements.

💰 You may be working for a local institution and receiving a local salary, or be given a small stipend for your time by an international organisation.

💰=0 If you go with an organisation, many will cover most costs such as flights and accommodation but you will be giving your time for free.

–💰 You may be entirely self-funding (volunteering or on elective) and need to pay for all costs yourself.

Pensions

Whilst you are overseas, you will not usually pay into the NHS pension scheme and this will affect your final pension entitlement. Your membership is frozen whilst you're away, but you can restart paying contributions when you return. It is possible to make additional voluntary contributions or a lump sum to make up your lost contributions when you come back.

The UK government was offering pension support for public sector employees who volunteered with certain organisations, but this sadly has been discontinued. If you want to make contributions whilst you are away, then you will need what is referred to as a Section 7(2) Direction. This is covered in detail in Chapter 9.

Tax

After all the expenses, it can be a pleasant surprise to discover that you may be entitled to a tax rebate for your time away. Each situation is different—see Chapter 9 on how to claim.

National insurance contributions

If you're going away for more than one full tax year, then you may want to make voluntary National Insurance contributions for the time you're away. This will ensure that you're entitled to the full State Pension and other bereavement benefits. However, both men and women now only need 30 qualifying years for the basic State Pension, so you may not need to make up short periods overseas in an otherwise long working life. See Chapter 9 for more details.

Electives

There's no way round it: an elective is going to cost you. Although you will be working, you're essentially going on an extended holiday for 2–3 months, and you need to budget accordingly. Unlike a holiday, however, there are ways to recoup some of the costs of an elective. Remember to start applying early and cast your net wide—you'll be surprised at the sources of possible funding. See Chapter 7 for funding ideas.

Family

The length of healthcare training can mean that the first chance you have to go away is after you have settled into a long-term relationship or had children. Alternatively, you may have only become interested in international work later on in your career, when you have suitable skills and experience that you now feel able to share.

Your family does not necessarily need to be a deterrent to your dreams, but you will need to make more arrangements and plan carefully. They will also influence what type of placement you decide to undertake and where you go.

Your partner

Essentially the choice is to go:

- on your own
- with your partner, who will
  - work with the same organisation or institution
  - work with a different organisation or institution
  - not work

If you decide to go without your partner, then you should choose your type of work and destination carefully. Placements can be in isolated or rural areas with non-existent or poor communications. Have you discussed how you will maintain your relationship during long periods with little contact? What is the cost of a flight home? Nearly all medium- and long-term placements allow periods of leave when your partner can come out or you can fly home. In addition, humanitarian organisations provide regular breaks (called 'R&R'—rest and recuperation) and make concessions for married couples.

If you decide to go together and both work, finding suitable employment in the same location before you go can be difficult. Some organisations will try to place you both together, but this will take longer if you are from different professional backgrounds. Opportunities are much more likely to arise *in situ*, so once one of you finds a good post in advance, the other might accept looking for opportunities on arrival.

If your partner decides to come but not work, then some organisations (e.g. VSO) do provide health insurance and other benefits for both people.

"I moved out to Malawi with my husband, who had arranged a post as an orthopaedic surgeon. I didn't initially have a job out there. However, when we got out, I made contact with the local teaching hospital and started doing some paediatric work. The mortality rate in the paediatric ward really made me see the need for palliative care. I eventually went on to set up the first paediatric palliative care service in the country—something I would have never anticipated doing before I arrived."

Dr Vicky Lavy, Malawi

Children

Although daunting, taking your children abroad with you can be done. A childhood experience of a different culture can have long-lasting rewards, at the very least in terms of horizons, awareness and tolerance. Children are very adaptable and will settle into most environments with few problems and often a huge amount of glee.

"I spent my childhood in Nepal, where my father was working with the United Nations. It was idyllic. I attended the international school in Kathmandu and had friends from all different nationalities and religions. It gave me tolerance and empathy towards other people and cultures, which has stood me in good stead in my career."

Dr Kate Mandeville (author)

"We took our 8-month-old baby out to Malawi with us, and returned home 10 years later with three boys aged 10, 8 and 5. It was an absolutely brilliant place for children, and they are very proud of their African heritage. In fact, they regularly ask us why we had to come back to England, and why we couldn't have stayed in Malawi!"

Dr Vicky Lavy, Malawi

Children may limit your options as you will probably want to be in urban centres with access to international schools (which can be expensive) or local schools of a high standard. Other options are home schooling or correspondence courses. Adequate health facilities are another consideration, as infants and small children are particularly at risk from tropical illnesses.

Some research grants and consultancy posts will offer allowances for 'dependents'. This usually refers to a non-earning partner and any children under 16 who are going to move with you to the placement. Senior consultancy packages sometimes include UK boarding school fees and return flights during holidays.

Find out more

- The Council of International Schools (*http://www.cois.org*) provides accreditation for international schools around the world. You can find a directory of international schools in more than 100 countries on its website.

Elderly parents

When you're younger, it's hard to imagine being the main caregiver to your parents. But this time can come quickly, and the idea of leaving elderly or vulnerable parents to go off overseas can be untenable. Clearly each situation is different, but if your parents are currently independent, then the time to go might be now rather than later.

What are the alternatives?

Having read this chapter, you may feel that this may not be the right time for you to go overseas. However, there are plenty of alternative ways in which you can prepare for and support international work in the UK.

Train up

If you can't go away now, think about building up your skills for future international work. For example, diplomas in tropical medicine or nursing are requested for clinical placements by many recruiting organisations. Courses in public health are highly regarded. Getting the right skills will maximise the impact of your time abroad. See Appendix 3 for a list of courses.

Languages

Time invested in learning a language now will widen your options in the future. If you've already got a good standard, perfect it so you can work competently as a health professional. The more time spent now, the less time spent adjusting when you do go away.

UK work

Helping with the home section of a link or twinning programme can be very rewarding. Hosting link staff on training visits or helping organise reciprocal trips will also increase your international experience.

Finally, there are many UK-based NGOs that need volunteers. Any number of these may reflect your particular interests, and are a worthwhile way of contributing to global campaigns. Chapter 15 describes further ways to get involved in international efforts whilst in the UK.

Conclusion

After reading this chapter, you should be in a good position to decide whether to remain in the UK for now or to look seriously into arranging time overseas. You should also have a good idea of the length of placement that is most suitable for your situation.

If the time is right for you, then the next section describes the types of work available, how to choose a location, and the practicalities of arranging and preparing for a placement.

REFERENCE

Miranda JJ, Yudkin JS, Willott C (2005). Global health electives: four years of experience. *Travel Medicine and Infectious Disease* 3(3):133–41.

Making it happen

The previous section introduced you to some of the global challenges and inequalities in health. You should now have an understanding of the role you, as an individual or part of an organisation, can play in this equation. You will have been able to analyse your motivations for doing international work and think about what you can really offer. If you are still reading, then you are ready to make international health work a reality in your career. This section will take you through the practical steps needed to achieve this, from first contact to packing your suitcase.

Chapter 5 (What work could you do?) summarises the different types of work that are available in international health. It will allow you to tailor your search to the most suitable placements.

Chapter 6 (Where could you work?) is an overview of the different regions of the world where you could work and the factors to consider in your choice of location.

Chapter 7 (Planning your placement) then runs you through how to arrange your placement, either on your own or through an organisation. It contains a directory of the most popular recruiting organisations.

Chapter 8 (Humanitarian relief) looks at emergency relief more closely, including how to get into the sector.

Finally, **Chapter 9 (Before you go)** gets down to the practicalities of preparing for your time abroad, both for work and for living away from home.

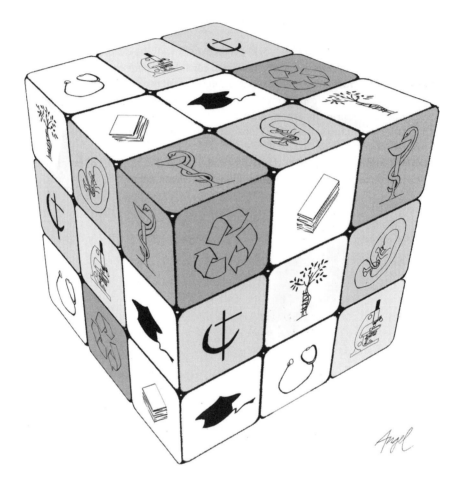

CHAPTER 5

What work could you do?

If you are reading on from Section 1, you have hopefully been now inspired. You have come to the conclusion that international work is possible for you. Now you can enter the exciting stage of deciding what you actually want to do overseas.

This process will be guided by your skills, temperament and attitude to risk. Be honest with yourself as this will lead to a much more successful placement than one where you've been overoptimistic about what you can cope with.

This chapter gives an overview of the broad categories of international health work available. Be aware that these are necessarily arbitrary. Many roles will involve a combination of several categories. For example, clinical practice will usually encompass an element of teaching.

Main types of global health work

- Humanitarian relief
- Rehabilitation/Development
- Clinical practice
- Student electives
- Teaching
- Research
- Consultancy

Other types of work that provide opportunities overseas are expedition and Armed Forces medicine. These are beyond the scope of this book, but there are plenty of resources available for those who are interested in these avenues into international work.

> **Find out more**
> ....
> **Armed forces medicine**
>
> - Ministry of Defence Careers. *http://www.mod.uk/defenceinternet/defencefor/jobseekers/*
> - *The Military Doctor*. Stephenson J. BMJ Career Focus 6.01.2010. **DOI:** 10.1136/bmj.b5437
> - *Training for the Front Line*. Randall-Carrick J. BMJ Career Focus 30.10.10. **DOI:** 10.1136/bmj.c5692
>
> **Expedition medicine**
>
> - Wilderness Medical Society. *http://www.wms.org*
> - Expedition Medicine training courses. *http://www.expeditionmedicine.co.uk/*
> - Diploma in Remote and Offshore Medicine, Royal College of Surgeons of Edinburgh. *http://www.diprom.rcsed.ac.uk*

Humanitarian relief

> **What does it involve?**
> ....
> - Short notice for departures
> - Short to medium term placements (<1 to 6 months)
> - Providing emergency treatment and restoring local services
> - Intense work in a cross-cultural team
> - Unstable and potentially dangerous conditions

Humanitarian relief work is initiated by crisis situations such as natural disasters, disease epidemics and conflicts. Local health services are often overwhelmed, and outside help is requested to cope with the number of people in need.

If you choose this type of work, you may end up working at short notice in very difficult conditions, usually whilst the situation is still unstable. You will be providing emergency treatment, maintaining essential services (such as maternity) and helping to restore local infrastructure.

This work is demanding, both physically and psychologically. You should be able to manage stress, work well in a team under difficult circumstances and cope well with arduous living conditions. This type of work is certainly not for everyone.

WHO SHOULD DO IT?

It really depends on the type of crisis. In the early stages of a crisis, very experienced people are needed. In the advent of a natural disaster, alongside a management team, there is a particular need for surgeons, anaesthetists and nephrologists (crush injuries from earthquakes often lead to renal failure). Clinical staff with experience in emergency medicine, surgery, paediatrics and obstetrics will be needed throughout the crisis.

For disease outbreaks such as cholera and measles, there will be a need for public health specialists. Mental health specialists may also be needed, particularly in violent locations.

As the crises settle down, relief organisations sometimes recruit people slightly less experienced to work under the guidance of others with more experience. Allied health professionals with particular management skills (for example pharmacists with medicine management experience) may be requested during the acute crisis, but this is less common. Therapists, both physical and psychological, will be needed more as the crisis draws to a close and aid efforts turn to rehabilitation.

Health professionals will need a minimum of 2 years' post-qualification experience. The intense nature of the work demands robust clinical skills, with little time for supervision.

Some people choose to pursue a full-time career in humanitarian relief, usually through permanent positions in relief organisations. These positions are limited, but you tend to receive a substantial amount of training as the organisation will see you as an investment.

WHAT SKILLS ARE DESIRABLE?

A diploma in tropical medicine or nursing is very useful, as is public health training. Further skills and training are outlined in Chapter 8.

"My work has often taken me to war zones like Sudan, Chad and the Congo. I am now Merlin's Reproductive Health Coordinator in Haiti, which has the highest maternal, infant and child mortality rates in the region. There were just 90 professionally trained midwives prior to the earthquake and the main midwifery school was badly damaged in the disaster. In my first month in the field, I performed 37 consultations on pregnant women, giving each a proper birth plan so they knew as much as possible about pregnancy and the childbirth process before going through it. We're also providing essential healthcare in underserved communities, supporting national health centres and helping earthquake survivors as they rebuild their lives. Although the work is demanding, I have the great fortune to be working with a highly motivated national team, which has made my work really enjoyable. I'm more passionate about my job than ever before."

Midwife, Haiti

Find out more
....

- Chapters 8 and 11 (and organisation websites listed in Chapter 7)
- *An Imperfect Offering: Humanitarian Action in the Twenty-first Century.* Orbinski J. Toronto: Doubleday Canada Written by the former head of MSF about his experiences in Rwanda and Somalia
- *War Games: The Story of Aid and War in Modern Times.* Polman L. New York: Viking. Journalist argues that humanitarian interventions prolong conflict, using examples of her experiences in Africa and Asia

Rehabilitation/Development

What does it involve?
....

- Medium- to long-term placements (several months to > 1 year)
- Organising services, managing projects, training local staff
- Working with local partners and communities
- Can involve living in rural/remote areas with minimal support
- Building local capacity and providing on-the-job training

This type of work focuses on long-term improvements in health outcomes and strengthening health systems. Rehabilitation concentrates on restoring health services after a crisis situation, helping the physical and psychological recovery of those affected, and the transition back to relative normality. Some humanitarian organisations also work in this area. It may lack the adrenaline of relief work, but it can be more satisfying in terms of producing sustained solutions.

Development work encompasses a wide spectrum of projects. In general, it aims to strengthen weak and fragile health systems, through capacity building and systems development. This is different to the 'gap-filling' of clinical practice. In fact, an indicator of the success of your work is making yourself redundant by training local people sufficiently to take on your post.

WHO SHOULD DO IT?

All health workers are suited to this type of work. Mental health professionals and therapists are needed in rehabilitation, and managers and public health practitioners have ideal skills for development projects.

WHAT SKILLS ARE DESIRABLE?

At least several years' professional experience and post-graduate qualifications in tropical medicine or public health are useful. Shorter training courses are listed in Appendix 3. Teaching skills are very useful as most projects will involve training local staff to improve capacity.

"I spent 2 years in northern Namibia as a Programme Adviser for an HIV/AIDS community-based NGO. We trained volunteers to be home-based care givers and ran a programme for orphaned and vulnerable children which included a hot meal, constructive play, help with school work and distributing free school uniforms. We also developed 'friend-ship clubs' where people who were HIV positive could give each other support and supported communities to develop their own agricultural and income generation projects. A great deal of our work was around community engagement and reducing stigma. We also worked closely with the health service as antiretroviral drugs were becoming more available so we were developing ways that our volunteers could support people on treatment.

My role was to build capacity in the organisation so included training staff on everything from basic project management skills, writing funding proposals and reports to using a computer and answering the phone. I even gave one member of staff some driving lessons!"

NHS manager, Namibia

Find out more

- Chapters 11 and 13 (and organisation websites listed in Chapter 7)
- Eliminating World Poverty: Building our Common Future (White Paper). DFID, 2009. *http://www.dfid.gov.uk/documents*
- *Working Effectively in Conflict-Affected and Fragile Situations* (series of briefing papers). DFID, 2010. *http://www.dfid.gov.uk/documents*
- The USAID-funded project CapacityPlus (*http://www.capacityplus.org/*) focuses on capacity building in the health workforce

Clinical practice

What does it involve?

- Short-, medium- and long-term placements
- Managing diseases and running services
- Working with and training local personnel
- Often a high workload and little supervision
- Frequent lack of resources

This is the most traditional type of international health work. Here, you may be filling an empty post, providing an extra pair of hands for an overloaded service or bringing your specialist skills to help those in need. Your role will focus on service provision, including teaching local colleagues. 'Pure' clinical posts are less common these days as the trend is for many organisations to move away from direct service delivery and towards building local capacity.

Clinical work overseas makes a contribution towards reversing the health worker crisis in poor countries. Although it may not solve the long-term problem, it undoubtedly helps those patients who would otherwise not have been treated. Host clinicians also cite the benefits of having overseas colleagues, including knowledge transfer and increased morale. However, it is worth thinking about the sustainability of your post. What will happen when you leave? In particular, what will happen to any services or systems that you have set up? See Chapter 13 for a fuller discussion.

WHO SHOULD DO IT?

All clinical staff.

WHAT SKILLS ARE DESIRABLE?

- At least 2–3 years' post-qualification experience
- Some training in tropical medicine/infectious diseases (particularly HIV/AIDS and TB)
- Management, supervision and training skills
- Ability to manage and prioritise high workload
- Improvisation in order to deal with lack of resources

"My first trip to Sierra Leone was purely clinical. I spent just over a week in a hospital identified by our local partner, an NGO. They sent out an appeal via the local radio for locals with symptoms of a hernia. A lot of people turned up on the first day, but luckily so did two junior doctors from the capital Freetown to help out. They triaged the patients, while I got on with the operating. About 90% turned out to be hernias, although one chap turned out to have acute appendicitis! I operated every day for a week in very hot conditions, as well as doing ward rounds and pre-operative assessment. At the time, there was only one clinical health officer at the hospital, who was probably doing most interventions. There was no anaesthetist so the theatre nurse used ketamine or local anaesthetic that I had brought out for spinal anaesthesia. Some patients were operated on under local anaesthetic alone, much as we do at home, although many of the hernias were too large for me easily to do this way."

Consultant surgeon, Sierra Leone

- Chapters 11 and 13 (and organisation websites listed in Chapter 7).
- *Where There Is No Doctor* (2nd edition). Werner D, Thuman C, Maxwell J. Hesperian, 1992. This classic manual was primarily intended for village health workers; however, it is highly valued by clinicians in LMIC for its concise and practical information. It has been translated into over 100 languages. There are now several sister manuals, including *Where There Is No Psychiatrist*.
- *Principles of Medicine in Africa* (3rd edition). Parry E, Godfrey R, Mabey D, Gill G (eds). Cambridge University Press, 2004.
- *Life After Injury: A Rehabilitation Manual for the Injured and their Helpers*. Hobbs L, McDonough S, O'Callaghan A. Third World Network, 2002.

Student electives

Medical students and some nursing students can undertake an elective period in another country as part of their training. Other trainee allied health professionals have taken electives, but this is not usually part of their formal training.

WHO SHOULD DO IT?

All trainee healthcare professionals who have the opportunity.

WHAT SKILLS ARE DESIRABLE?

- Languages
- Initiative and self-directed learning
- Self-sufficiency
- Respect for different cultures
- Awareness of limits of competency

"I spent 8 weeks in Guyana on my elective in the fifth year of medical school. I worked in the emergency department of a hospital in the capital. Primary healthcare was pretty much non-existent so I was seeing a lot more advanced pathology than I had in the UK. There was also a lot of violence and I saw many gunshot wounds.

Patients were very deferential to doctors and expected them to be omnipotent, which meant taking a history could be very frustrating. Open-ended questions were not that useful, as most patients wouldn't elaborate. Sometimes they would just reply, 'You're the healer—you tell me!' Almost all of the patients had no clue about their past medical history. There was a strong culture of paternalism which meant the patients would often be

➲

given drugs or treatments without the diagnosis being explained or even told to them. I had been told it was an English-speaking country—in fact, the only one in Latin America, which is why I chose it. However, when I got there, I realised the English was in fact pidgin English, which might as well be a different language. The terminology used by the patients was very different and a nurse had to stay with me during my histories at first to translate. For example, 'I've got sugar' meant that they were diabetics who had had a positive urine dipstick for glucose.

I found a couple of things difficult. Firstly, there was a very different attitude towards sharps safety and infection control. This was partly because of a lack of resources (e.g. gloves) but also due to a lack of awareness of hospital-acquired infections, whereas it's drummed into us in the UK. I also didn't like the treatment of indigenous Amerindian patients, as they received very obvious discrimination from the medical staff."

Emergency doctor, Guyana

Find out more

- See Elective Advice and 'You Pay' section in Chapter 7. Also Chapters 11 and 13
- *Therapy Elective Overseas*. Christian Medical Fellowship, 2004. *http://www.cmf. org.uk/internationalministries/electives.asp*
- Guidance on Planning an Elective at Home or Overseas. BMA Medical Students Committee, 2009
- Ethics and Medical Electives in Resource-Poor Countries—a Toolkit. BMA, 2009. Read this in conjunction with the above guide
- *Beyond Borders: McGraw-Hill's Guide to Health Placements*. Graham H. McGraw-Hill, 2005

Teaching

What does it involve?

- Short-, medium- and long-term placements
- Training health workers in your particular skills
- Either on-the-job or formal lecturing at health worker training institutions.
- Needs careful evaluation to show impact and transfer of knowledge from theory to practice.

Most clinical and rehabilitation/development roles will contain an element of informal teaching, but there is also a high demand for full-time clinical teachers. Recent initiatives to massively scale up the numbers of trained health workers mean that many countries do not have sufficient teaching staff to deliver these goals. Health training institutions are frequently short-staffed and may lack expertise in specific areas. Filling these gaps can be very rewarding work and can be arranged directly with the institution you are supporting, if your skills meet their needs.

Short-term visits can easily be incorporated into annual leave, and many individuals do this on a regular basis. It is vital to arrange these visits well in advance and ensure your visit corresponds with the time frame for delivery of the curriculum. Many people build up a relationship and return as external examiners.

While these short-term placements can be useful, longer-term teaching posts are often more valued by the partner institution. If you cannot commit to this yourself, you might be prepared to organise a rolling programme of visits, by different lecturers or examiners, for longer periods of time.

Teaching is one of the most sustainable ways to use your skills in resource-poor environments, and is often specifically requested by overseas partners. An increasing trend is for 'train the trainers' courses: a core group of health workers are trained in a technique, who then go on to teach it to their colleagues, and so on. An important aspect of all training is the need for robust evaluation—can you show that your teaching is having an impact?

WHO SHOULD DO IT?

All health workers, including healthcare scientists and managers. However, do double-check that the audience and curriculum are appropriate for your level.

WHAT SKILLS ARE DESIRABLE?

Previous teaching experience is a bonus, especially for shorter visits. This way you will know what works and be able to hit the ground running. However, all the best laid plans will need adjusting for cultural differences and unexpected problems.

Previous involvement in setting examinations or course evaluation would also be useful, as would curriculum development and examining. At some point, you are likely to have to justify your trip to someone. You will be in a much stronger position to do this with evidence of improved knowledge or skills, for example through validated pre- and post-course tests.

"In 2006 Malawi only had one qualified psychiatrist, who was singlehand-edly responsible for mental health services in Malawi and teaching undergraduate medical students. On my first contact with the College of Medicine it was clear that supporting undergraduate teaching in psychiatry was essential to improve the mental health services in the country.

➔

Working with a small group of interested colleagues, we founded the Scotland—Malawi Mental Health Education Project (http://www.smmhep.org.uk). For each of the last 3 years, we have sent up to seven Scottish trainees in psychiatry to the College of Medicine. They spend 6–8 weeks delivering theory and clinical teaching to the fourth-year medical students. The project is well supported by the volunteers' employers and many are allowed special leave accredited for training purposes and continue to receive their basic salaries whilst they are in Malawi.

The structured nature of the curriculum means that the volunteers don't need to have had a lot of teaching experience beforehand. Student feedback on the quality of their teaching has been very positive. As we have an agreed structure, disruption to the local institution is minimal. Our work will ensure that the future leaders of Malawi's health service will have a sound understanding of mental healthcare, which has until now been largely neglected."

Psychiatrist, Malawi

Find out more

....

- Chapters 11 and 13
- *What Difference Are We Making? A Toolkit on Monitoring and Evaluation for Health Links.* Gordon M, Potts C. Tropical Health and Education Trust, 2008. *http://www.thet.org.uk*

Research

What does it involve?

....

- Usually medium- and long-term placements
- Self-directed work which requires persistence and diplomacy
- Results may have little impact on practice
- Competitive funding

The UK has a strong history of research into tropical medicine and international health. There are many excellent institutions in the UK where it is perfectly possible to follow an academic career in global health. Although short projects are available, most studies will require longer placements.

Organising research in resource-poor countries can be very different to in the UK. Ethics committees can be difficult to track down and very slow, and often delay or even derail projects. Cultural misunderstandings can threaten the validity of results, so it is often worth liaising with local staff during data collection. However, research capacity is usually low, so you may need to factor in training time and costs. Dealing with local officials can require a great deal of diplomacy to sort out logistical details. Due to these differences, it is always worth seeking out a supervisor or advisory panel with experience in low-income countries until you gain enough experience.

WHO SHOULD DO IT?

All health workers with an academic interest.

WHAT SKILLS ARE DESIRABLE?

- Initiative and motivation
- Diplomacy and negotiation skills
- Research skills, e.g. specialist software or epidemiology
- Previous experience in LMIC

"I spent my elective in Peru carrying out research into the cost-effectiveness of expanding their HIV programmes. My Peruvian supervisor had carried out a lot of research out there previously so knew the system well. I did as much work as I could before I left, so I could concentrate on data collection when I was out there. It was pretty inspiring working with these amazing Peruvian researchers who were also outstanding clinicians. When I came back, I continued data analysis with regular Skype and email contact with the team out there. You have to be very disciplined about writing up, otherwise it's very easy to let things slide once you're back at home. The paper was published last year, and it was really satisfying to see it finally out there. One of the best things about Peru was making contact with another research group there, for whom I am now doing the analysis of a novel tuberculosis diagnostic test."

Academic clinician, Peru

Find out more

- Chapters 11 and 12
- Two major UK funding bodies for research into tropical medicine and global health are the Wellcome Trust (*http://www.wellcome.ac.uk*) and the Medical Research Council (*http://www.mrc.ac.uk*). Their websites provide details on their various fellowship and funding schemes.

- Although many UK universities do health research overseas, it's worth regularly checking the vacancy pages of those that concentrate on tropical medicine and global health, including:
  - London School of Hygiene and Tropical Medicine (*http://www.lshtm.ac.uk*)
  - Liverpool School of Tropical Medicine (*http://www.liv.ac.uk*)
  - UCL Institute for Global Health (*http://www.ucl.ac.uk/global-health/*)
  - Nuffield Centre for International Health and Development (*http://www.leeds.ac.uk/nuffield/*)

Advisory/Consultancy

What does it involve?

- Usually short- and medium-term placements
- Using your specialist skills to advise or manage projects
- High degree of technical competence necessary
- Little job security
- Frequent applications necessary for new assignments

Consultancy work is another excellent way to impart your skills to partners in global health. The level of input varies by project: you may be advising on just a certain aspect, or you may manage the whole project yourself.

This type of work is realistically only available to those with specialist skills or extensive experience. Contacts are extremely important in identifying new assignments, and you could also register your profile with governmental organisations, NGOs and other consultancy firms (see Appendix 1). You will need to submit your proposal in response to calls advertised on agency websites. If you go into it full time, consider registering yourself as a company or self-employed, which can assist with tax relief.

WHO SHOULD DO IT?

Senior professionals and/or those with niche skills.

WHAT SKILLS ARE DESIRABLE?

- Ability to manage several projects at once—you may be combining this work with some NHS work or other projects in the UK
- A high level of technical knowledge
- Previous experience at international level

- Diplomacy and cross-cultural skills—you will usually be working in a multicultural team and often dealing with government officials
- Languages

"Becoming a consultant after having been a chief executive was a steep learning curve. I had to learn new skills particularly relating to managing my time, logistics and IT. I was working simultaneously in different countries and had to understand their social, institutional and political structures and disease profiles.

Most work is undertaken in partnership. This means working with Ministries of Health, with bilateral and multilateral organisations and NGOs such as BRAC in Bangladesh and the Health Systems Trust in South Africa. Increasingly one is working with the private sector including the pharmaceutical industry. My work has been very varied, but has tended to focus on strategic planning, health workforce issues, organisational development and evaluations. The work is rewarding, very challenging and diverse. I continue to learn a lot.

The market for consultants has changed in the last 15 years. It is probably smaller now than 10 years ago as countries have developed their own capacity and only people with specialist knowledge together with broad development experience are needed. For people who do not have a development background it is becoming increasingly difficult to get recruited, as health in a developed country setting is very different to a low-income setting. In the past, much of the work was in relatively stable countries. Increasingly the requests are coming from post-conflict countries such as Iraq, Afghanistan, Sudan and so on. We are having to learn a new context from this experience because it means that geopolitics of aid, health development and security are becoming linked and this is a new dimension of the job."

International health consultant

Find out more

- See 'Career Opportunities' section of Chapter 7 and Chapter 15
- *A Core Competency Framework for International Health Consultants*. World Health Professions Alliance (WHPA), 2007. *http://www.whpa.org*
- The vacancy pages of the WHO often call for consultants in specialist areas and it's worth checking this regularly. Organisations such as the British Executive Service Overseas (which merged with VSO in 2006) offer short-term specialist assignment or senior consultants for troubleshooting roles. To become involved in these you generally have to be senior in your role and have had previous experience of this type of work
- For fledgling consultants, the short course in International Health Consultancy offered by LSTM may be of interest. More details are given in Appendix 3
- HMRC has an excellent guide for those starting out in business explaining all the major issues, such as tax, National Insurance and record keeping. They will send you the guide automatically if you register as self-employed with them

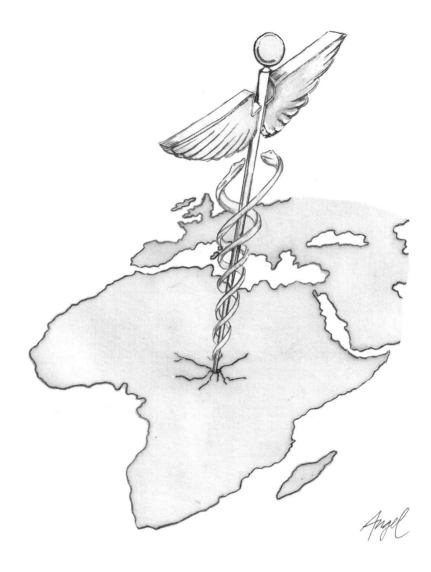

Angel

CHAPTER 6

Where could you work?

One of the most exciting aspects of planning a period of work overseas is deciding your destination. How will you make your choice? In this chapter, we give an overview of world regions where you are likely to be working and what might influence your decision.

If you are arranging your own placement, your destination is largely under your control. Remember, however, that an organisation must send you to their priority zones.

The first part of this chapter looks at the factors to consider in more detail, while the second part illustrates each of these factors by region. Generalisations have been made for the sake of clarity, so once you know which country you will be working in, do read up on its health system and health indicators in more detail. The country profiles available on the WHO website are a good start (http://www.who.int/countries/en/).

Factors to consider when selecting a destination

- Languages
- Risk of conflict
- Health needs
- Health worker shortage
- Climate
- Personal health risks

Languages

It may come as a surprise that only a dozen or so countries throughout the world use English as their common language.

Of course, the legacy of colonisation has meant that many countries have a European language as one of their official languages. However, most countries also have a bewildering array of local languages and the *lingua franca* is likely only to be the domain of the educated. Even then, it will often only be their second or third language.

There are nearly 7,000 languages spoken in the world today, a fact that is difficult to comprehend for us relatively mono-linguistic Europeans (see Table 6.1). Papua New Guinea has nearly 10% (820) of these, an average of 7,000 speakers per language. Indonesia (737), Nigeria (510) and India (415) also have a large number of native languages. At the other end of the scale, Belarus, the Maldives, Rwanda and the Democratic People's Republic of Korea each have only one indigenous living language (Lewis 2009).

Table 6.1 Estimated number of languages spoken in different regions of the world

Asia	2240
Africa	2100
The Pacific	1330
The Americas	1050
Europe	210

Fluency in at least one of the official languages of a country is an essential prerequisite and will be a major factor limiting your choice of destination. If you are lucky enough to be bi- or even tri-lingual, then many other countries will open up to you (see Figure 6.1).

Remember that whilst you may be able to speak to your Togolese colleagues in French, many of your patients (and support staff) will only speak local dialects. Fluency in local languages will be an advantage and if you are in a long-term post it will help you enormously if you make an effort to learn it. Some organisations do offer language training. Constantly requiring a translator can be a drain on local resources, and negate the positive impact of your visit.

"I chose to do my elective in Bolivia because I had a contact who knew a Bolivian GP and he helped me to set up my first placement. I didn't speak Spanish so I spent 6 weeks at a language school and another 6 weeks working in a clinic in the city. I loved the place and went back on several short visits. I then returned for a year after my foundation programme and started by doing another 6 weeks at the language school."

Junior doctor, Bolivia

Find out more

....

- Lonely Planet publishes phrasebooks in a number of indigenous languages, e.g. Thai and Quechua. Digital and mobile versions are also available and NHS employees can get a discount. http://shop.lonelyplanet.com/phrasebooks
- The American Peace Corps produces some excellent language guides for their volunteers. Some of these are available online. Try a Google search for American Peace Corps language guide and the name of the local language.
- Try to track down a medical textbook or dictionary in the dominant language before your departure.

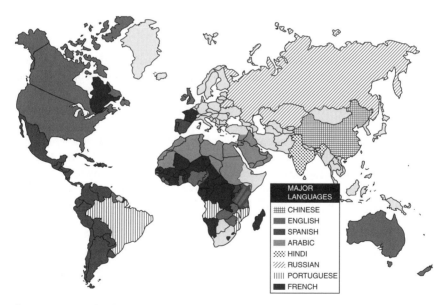

Figure 6.1 Major languages of the world. (Maps courtesy of http://www.theodora.com/maps, used with permission).

If you are going with an organisation and have indicated that you speak another language, they are likely to test your fluency during the interview. If you are arranging your own placement, it is up to you to assess whether your level is sufficient. Your GCSE French may be adequate for exchanging pleasantries, but are you really able to ask someone to pass the scalpel? Of course, there is nothing like being in the country itself for improving your language skills. However, it is your responsibility to ensure that your level of language is adequate to function in stressful clinical situations before you leave (see Box 6.1). This could be through personal language lessons tailored to medical terminology, or joining an association such as the Anglo-French Medical Society, which holds regular meetings on medical topics (http://www.anglofrenchmedical.org).

Box 6.1: To think about

Ask yourself honestly—do you have the level of fluency needed to operate in a different healthcare system? For example, would you be able to:
• Ask for surgical instruments during an operation?
• Take an accurate history from a patient?
• Direct a resuscitation team?
• Write a situation report?
• Negotiate with Ministry of Health officials on complex issues?

Risk of conflict

There were over 30 recognised conflicts in the world occurring at the time of writing. Many have been ongoing for decades. The website http://www.globalsecurity.org gives a list of current world conflicts.

If you choose to work in these zones, the risk of harm is very real. While International Humanitarian Law protects medical personnel, a review of deaths of medical humanitarian workers found that intentional violence was the cause in 57% of cases between 1985 and 1998 (Sheik *et al.* 2000). Between 2006 and 2008, 75% of attacks on aid workers occurred in just seven countries, the most dangerous being Sudan, Afghanistan and Somalia (Hill *et al.* 2010). If you do choose to work with a humanitarian organisation in a conflict zone, security will be one of their prime concerns. Ultimately, you must make a personal risk assessment of the situation and decide if you are comfortable with that level of risk.

Conflict zones tend to have very acute health needs. In the countries with the ten highest rates of maternal deaths, nine are either at war or emerging from conflict (Merlin 2010). Similarly, 22 of the 34 countries furthest from achieving the MDGs are in or recovering from conflict (DFID 2007). International health workers make a huge difference in these areas by supporting or providing a local health service, and many populations would be even worse off if these workers didn't accept the associated risks.

In the regional overview below, we have used the Global Peace Index (GPI) to give you an indication of the stability of a country (http://www.visionofhumanity.org). The GPI ranks countries by their 'absence of violence' using metrics that combine both internal and external factors. It is composed of 23 indicators, ranging from a nation's level of military expenditure to its relations with neighbouring countries and the level of respect for human rights, using data collated by the Economist Intelligence Unit. Lower scores indicate a more peaceful country.

Health needs

Another major factor that should influence your choice is the relative health needs of a country. Where will your skills make the most difference? Which countries need you most?

The starkest indicator of need is mortality rates. WHO has divided its 192 member states into five mortality strata on the basis of their mortality rates for children under 5 years of age and men aged 15–59 years (see Table 6.2). This gives a good indication of the health status of each country and we include the mortality stratum for each member country in the regional overviews below.

Table 6.2 World Health Organization mortality strata

WHO mortality stratum	Child mortality (C)	Adult mortality (A)	Abbreviation
A	Very low	Low	VLCLA
B	Low	Low	LCLA
C	Low	High	LCHA
D	High	High	HCHA
E	High	Very high	HCVHA

As described in Chapter 1, mortality rates don't tell you everything about the disease burden in a country. DALYs (the sum of years of potential life lost due to premature mortality and the years of productive life lost due to disability) are often used to give an estimate of the disease burden from different causes. This is usually divided into three broad causes:

- Communicable diseases, maternal and perinatal conditions, and nutritional deficiencies
- Non-communicable diseases
- Injuries

The ratio of disease burden by these three causes varies by region. This is likely to affect the types of projects available to you and which skills are most needed in each region. For example, health workers in sub-Saharan Africa are much more likely to be dealing with the prevention and treatment of communicable diseases than those in Eastern Europe (see Figure 6.2).

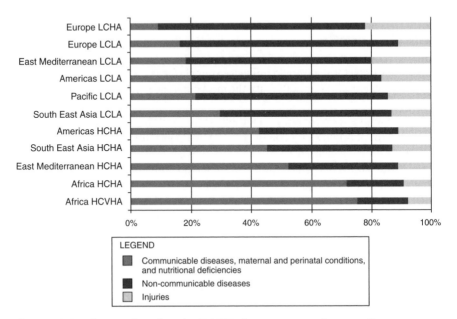

Figure 6.2 Disease burden in DALYs by cause and mortality stratum in WHO region (2002 estimates). Reproduced with kind permission of the WHO.

Another way of assessing the need for your skills would be by the number of health workers available for that country's population. Countries with fewer than 2.5 health workers (counting only doctors, nurses and midwives) per 1,000 population are defined as having a critical shortage. Figure 6.3 shows the distribution of the 57 countries assessed as having a critical shortage of health workers in 2006. Thirty-five of those countries are in sub-Saharan Africa. Further data on the health workforce for all UN member states can be found at the Global Health Observatory website (http://www.who.int/gho/en/).

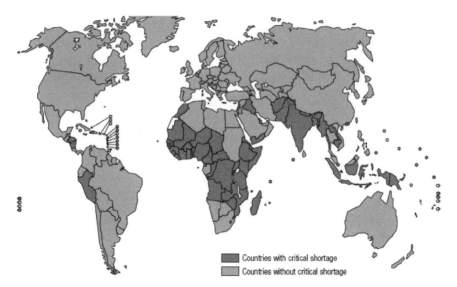

| | Countries with critical shortage |
| | Countries without critical shortage |

Figure 6.3 Countries with a critical shortage of health service providers (doctors, nurses and midwives). Reproduced with kind permission of the WHO (World Health Report 2006).

Climate

If you are arranging your own placement, you will have the luxury of selecting the type of climate to which you are most suited. Don't underestimate the sapping effect of heat and humidity on motivation and productivity. If you are not good in the sun or have a high-risk skin type, then consider focusing on countries with a more temperate climate (see Figure 6.4).

If you will be travelling to high altitudes, you must factor in time for acclimatisation. Altitude illness is a very real threat, and it is difficult to predict individual susceptibility in advance. Travel to altitudes above 3,500 m immediately from sea level should be avoided whenever possible. The most important prevention measures are gradual ascent to allow acclimatisation and regular rest days.

Find out more
....
- National Travel Health Network and Centre. *http://www.nathnac.org/travel/factsheets/altitude.htm*

Health considerations

The following factors probably won't dissuade you from an exciting placement, but they are worth bearing in mind if you are presented with a choice of posts.

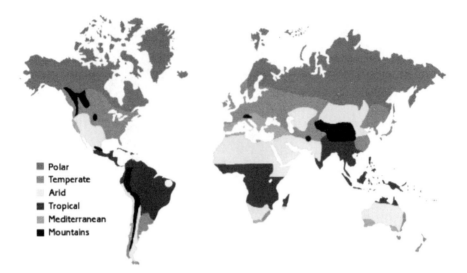

Figure 6.4 Map of world climate zones. © Crown copyright 2011, the met office.

Malaria chemoprophylaxis

If your placement is in a malarious zone, then you should take effective chemoprophylaxis for all of this time, as well as preventing bites. This can have side effects and be expensive. If your placement is medium or long term and you have had side effects on antimalarials before, then this may influence your choice of region (see Figure 6.5).

Blood-borne viruses

If you are going to be performing many invasive procedures, then be aware of the local prevalence of blood-borne viruses such as hepatitis B, hepatitis C and HIV. Prevalence is likely to be higher in areas where health needs are particularly acute. In these settings, scrupulous infection control measures and availability of post-exposure prophylaxis (PEP) are essential.

Road traffic accidents

WHO estimates that 1.2 million people are killed and 20–50 million people are injured worldwide every year as a result of road traffic accidents. Most of these deaths and injuries occur in LMIC. If you are likely to be driving or using vehicles regularly as part of your work, make sure you read the preparation section in Chapter 9 and the driving abroad page on the FCO website (http://www.fco.gov.uk).

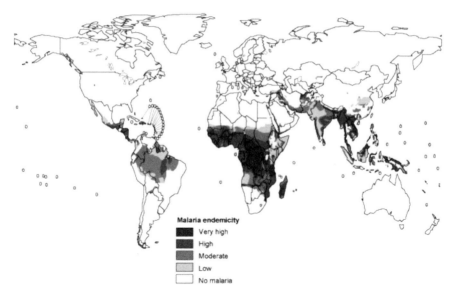

Figure 6.5 Map of global distribution of malaria transmission risk, 2003. Reproduced with kind permission of the WHO (WHO Malaria Report 2005).

Overview of regions

We have arranged countries into groupings based on proximity, climate and disease burden. These groupings broadly follow the WHO regions, but not completely. Each regional map includes the GPI for countries where available and the WHO mortality strata. This should give you a good introduction to each region, which can be followed up by more specific country reading.

> **Find out more**
>
> ....
>
> - *WHO Regional Office websites* (listed below by region). Provides data, policies and health topics specific to that region
> - *WHO Country Profiles. http://www.who.int/gho/countries.* Contains vital health information from the Global Health Observatory for each WHO member state, including mortality and burden of disease, outbreaks, immunisation profile, and health financing and workforce
> - *The CIA World Factbook. http://www.cia.gov/library/publications/the-world-factbook.* Lists population, government, military and economic information for nations recognised by the United States

We've excluded countries with very low child and adult mortality (and their overseas territories) from this overview, in keeping with our focus on international health.

Central America

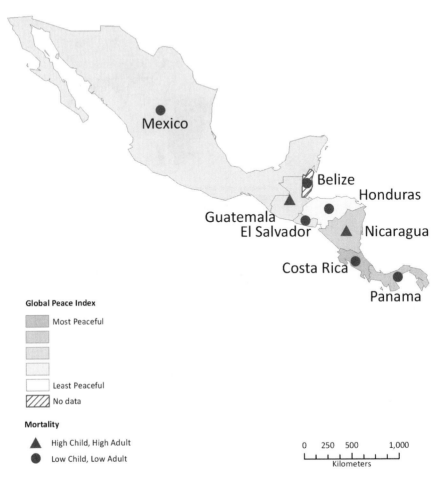

Global Peace Index

	Most Peaceful
	Least Peaceful
	No data

Mortality

▲ High Child, High Adult
● Low Child, Low Adult

0 250 500   1,000
Kilometers

OFFICIAL LANGUAGE(S)

Spanish, except:

- Guatemala = plus 23 officially recognised Amerindian languages
- Belize = official language English, but Spanish spoken widely
- Nicaragua = English spoken along Atlantic coast
- Panama = English spoken widely

"I spent 8 weeks working in a clinic and a hospital in Honduras during one of my summers at medical school. They were both in a very rural and poor area; the public clinic was run by an American charity and the hospital was part of the national health system. Both were very under-staffed and had few resources. Families used to have to bring in the sheets and food for their relatives who were in-patients in the hospital.

There was an epidemic of dengue fever when I arrived, and the junior doctors were overwhelmed by the work. I split my time mostly between the emergency department, the delivery room and the very sparse the-atre. After 3 weeks, a delegation of Cuban doctors arrived to help, which made a big difference to the workload.

My Spanish was pretty good, but it took me a few days to tune into the accent. Everyone was very pleased that I was talking Spanish, including my landlady who would take me out to the local disco! Most doctors could speak some English, but in order to communicate with the patients you had to speak Spanish so it's important to bear that in mind when deciding whether to go.

Central America is great for travelling in your free time, as the countries are so close together yet have very different identities. My husband came out at the end of my placement, and we travelled around for sev-eral weeks."

Medical student, Honduras

Find out more

- WHO regional office website: *http://www.paho.who.int*

The Caribbean

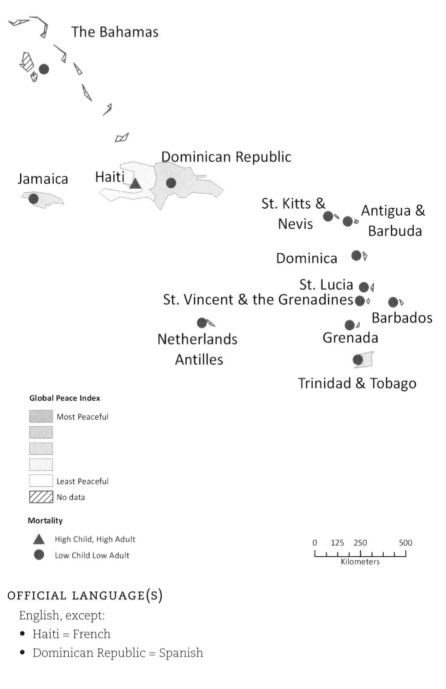

The Bahamas

Dominican Republic

Jamaica   Haiti

St. Kitts & Nevis

Antigua & Barbuda

Dominica

St. Lucia

St. Vincent & the Grenadines

Barbados

Netherlands Antilles

Grenada

Trinidad & Tobago

Global Peace Index

Most Peaceful

Least Peaceful

No data

Mortality

High Child, High Adult

Low Child Low Adult

0   125   250   500
Kilometers

OFFICIAL LANGUAGE(S)

English, except:

- Haiti = French
- Dominican Republic = Spanish

"I arrived in Haiti 4 days into the cholera epidemic of late 2010. Patient numbers were increasing and threatening to overwhelm local capacity. Our MSF team set up and ran a cholera treatment centre, expanding it as the epidemic grew over the next few weeks. I took the lead on many managerial issues, including recruitment of extra staff, organising rosters and discipline.

I had to conduct interviews and teach the nurses in French. All the nurses spoke classical French, whereas those patients who were less educated spoke only Creole. This is a very different language and I needed to ask Haitian nurses to translate for me for these patients.

I also used my background in intensive care and resuscitation to provide direct patient care when needed. Although it was tropical, I only really noticed this during emergency situations when it got very hot and sticky.

The expatriate staff lived in a house about 10–15 minutes drive from the hospital. After getting home from an 11-hour day, all we wanted to do was sit around talking on the balcony and going to bed early. I didn't really see much else of Haiti during my visit, as there was so much to do at work. I never felt personally vulnerable during my visit, but our MSF unit was very rigorous on security. For example, we were driven most places, and I can only remember walking a few metres in the street on one occasion.

Overall, it was really satisfying to put systems in place and see patient outcomes improve because of it."

Nurse, Haiti

Find out more

- WHO regional office website: *http://www.paho.who.int*

South America

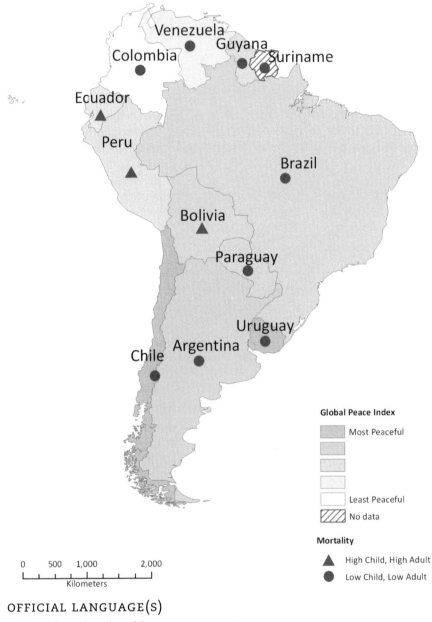

Venezuela
Colombia
Guyana
Suriname
Ecuador
Peru
Brazil
Bolivia
Paraguay
Uruguay
Argentina
Chile

Global Peace Index

Most Peaceful

Least Peaceful

No data

Mortality

▲ High Child, High Adult

● Low Child, Low Adult

0   500   1,000   2,000
Kilometers

OFFICIAL LANGUAGE(S)

Spanish and national languages, except:

- Brazil = Portuguese
- Surinam = Dutch, English, Hindi
- Guyana = English

"I spent my elective doing clinical work and research on HIV in Peru. I was based at the Institute of Tropical Medicine in Lima, which is renowned throughout South America. The clinicians and researchers were unbelievably good, and had incredible clinical skills. The hospital was very organised as they regularly received elective students. For example, I was put on a firm with two other students from Chile. Elective students weren't allowed to do any procedures though.

It was the first time I had worked in Spanish, and I was utterly exhausted at the end of every ward round. I got a lot better during the 3 months, but it was still pretty tough at the end. It was fine as an elective student, but it would have been difficult actually working as a doctor.

Lima itself was lovely, as it's fairly mild, despite being in the tropics and in the middle of a desert. The food in Peru is incredible, and was definitely a highlight. I would go back just for the food."

Academic clinician, Peru

Find out more

• WHO regional office website: *http://www.paho.who.int*

North Africa and the Middle East

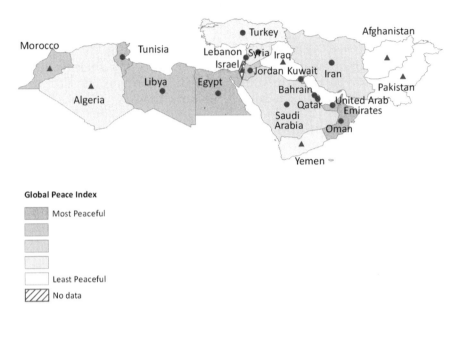

Global Peace Index

- Most Peaceful
-
-
-
- Least Peaceful
- No data

Mortality

- ▲ High Child, High Adult
- ● Low Child, Low Adult

0   750   1,500   3,000
Kilometers

OFFICIAL LANGUAGE(S)

Arabic and national languages, except:

- Sudan = plus English
- Djibouti = plus French
- Algeria, Lebanon, Morocco, Tunisia = French spoken widely
- Pakistan = Urdu and English

"I spent 6 weeks in South Sudan running an emergency 220-bed cholera camp during an outbreak. We had up to 80 admissions a day as well as numerous people who were observed for some time on oral fluids. The hospital was set up by MSF and run mostly by local clinical officers and nurses.

It was a tough environment. It was incredibly hot and dry and the hospital was essentially made up of large canvas tents which felt like a greenhouses. Communication with the local staff was not a problem, but it was sometimes more difficult with the foreign staff who were all Spanish. We didn't experience any violence, although there were reports of attacks in nearby areas.

I was amazed to see patients getting better within a few hours; however, the work was pretty relentless."

Paediatrician, Sudan

Find out more

....

• WHO regional office website: *http://www.emro.who.int*

Sub-Saharan and Southern Africa

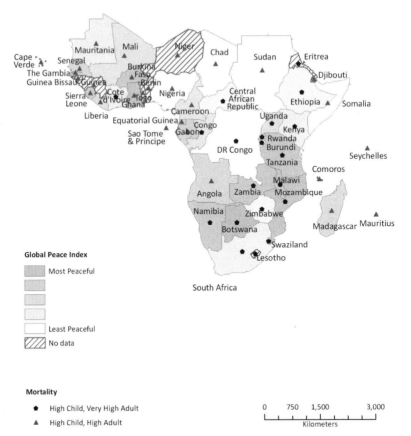

Global Peace Index

- Most Peaceful
-
-
-
- Least Peaceful
- No data

Mortality

- High Child, Very High Adult
- High Child, High Adult

0   750   1,500   3,000

Kilometers

OFFICIAL LANGUAGE(S)

National languages plus:

- Angola, Cape Verde, Guinea-Bissau, Mozambique, Sao Tome and Principe = Portuguese
- Benin, Burundi, Burkina Faso, Cameron, Central African Republic, Chad, Comoros, Congo, Côte d'Ivoire, Democratic Republic of the Congo, Gabon, Guinea, Madagascar, Mali, Mauritius, Niger, Rwanda, Senegal, Seychelles, Togo = French
- Botswana, Cameroon, Eritrea, the Gambia, Ghana, Kenya, Lesotho, Liberia, Malawi, Mauritius, Namibia, Nigeria, Rwanda, Seychelles, Sierra Leone, Swaziland, Tanzania, Uganda, Zambia, Zimbabwe = English
- Chad, Comoros, Eritrea, Mali, Mauritania = Arabic
- Equatorial Guinea = French and Spanish
- South Africa = 11 official languages, including Afrikaans and English

"I was based in Oshakati, the principal town in Northern Namibia. Everything was very hot and dusty and I felt like I was living in the middle of a desert. It was a little strange at first not to have access to large shopping centres, gyms, cinemas and other forms of entertainment. However, as there were other volunteers locally, we were able to make our own entertainment by sharing books and DVDs, playing volleyball and tennis, and attending local cultural events. It was nice to occasionally go to the capital Windhoek for a dose of Western culture!

At work the staff and volunteers were very welcoming. They would often sing and dance to greet me if I had been away. I did sometimes find it hard to have a constructive discussion about work issues as Namibians are quite deferential. Sometimes they would agree with me or say 'yes' to something because they thought that was what I wanted to hear.

Communication could be tricky. Although English is an official language, many women in the community spoke only their local language, Oshiwambo or Afrikaans. I often had to use staff members as translators. One of my favourite tasks was to present certificates to our newly-trained volunteer. I was keen to give my congratulatory speech in Oshiwambo so a colleague translated what I wanted to say. It is a very phonetic language so I learned to read it. I wasn't entirely sure of what I was saying but did get a huge round of applause at the end!"

NHS manager, Namibia

Find out more

....

• WHO regional office website: *http://www.afro.who.int*

Indian Subcontinent

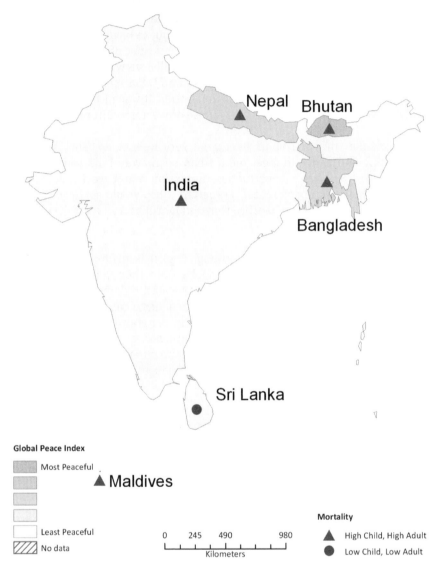

Global Peace Index
- Most Peaceful
- Least Peaceful
- No data

Mortality
- ▲ High Child, High Adult
- ● Low Child, Low Adult

Kilometers
0   245   490   980

OFFICIAL LANGUAGE(S)
India = Hindi and English, plus recognised regional languages
Others = national languages, but English spoken widely

"I spent 2 months at a hospital in Dharamsala in northern India. It's the seat of the exiled Tibetan government, and the hospital practised both Tibetan and Western medicine. I went with an open mind about Tibetan medicine, and saw a lot of interesting results.

The hospital ran on very similar lines to the NHS. It was very busy, and the staff were overworked and underpaid. Unsurprisingly, I spent a lot of time in TB outpatient clinics and on infectious disease management—despite having only two antibiotics to prescribe. There were also unexpected health needs. There were quite a lot of angry young male refugees in Dharamsala, and we dealt with quite a few drug and alcohol misuse problems. We also had an Indian psychiatrist who treated victims of torture.

The climate was perfect—it's at higher altitude so didn't get too hot, but could be cold at night. A drawback was that it was very touristy, although that meant that there were plenty of internet cafes and cheap restaurants around.

I came back to a placement in Whitechapel in London, and found myself applying many of the lessons I had learnt in Dharamsala."

Pharmacist, India

Find out more

• WHO regional office website: *http://www.searo.who.int*

South East Asia and the Far East

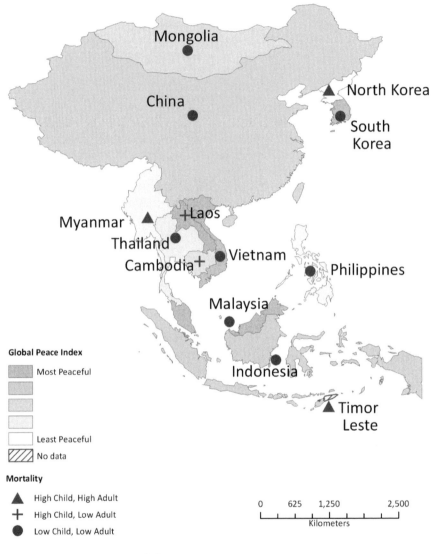

Global Peace Index

- Most Peaceful
- Least Peaceful
- No data

Mortality

- ▲ High Child, High Adult
- ✚ High Child, Low Adult
- ● Low Child, Low Adult

0   625   1,250   2,500
Kilometers

OFFICIAL LANGUAGE(S)

National languages, but Mandarin spoken widely

"I spent 3 months in Cambodia, working in a medical team made of three doctors and a midwife, me, at the Millennium Development Village (MDV) in Samlaut, northwest Cambodia. (*MDVs are projects that aim to increase capacity and community empowerment in Africa and Asia through training and knowledge sharing with local African and Asian governments, NGOs and village communities.*)

Language was definitely a barrier. We had to work with translators all the time, which I found restrictive. Working with women and having a male translator was not always appropriate. It also meant I tended to socialise with the UK team, rather than the local staff.

I found people in Cambodia very accepting, as they had been through a war and were emotionally flat. People appeared to live together in harmony, but unfortunately I wasn't able to get a deeper understanding of the conflict and its impact because of the language divide.

Luckily, we went during the dry season, so it wasn't too humid. It can be difficult to work during the rainy season because the heat can feel really oppressive as well as difficulties travelling to and from the headquarters of the MDV."

Midwife, Cambodia

Find out more

• WHO regional offices websites: *http://www.searo.who.int* and *http://www.wpro.who.int*

Pacific Islands

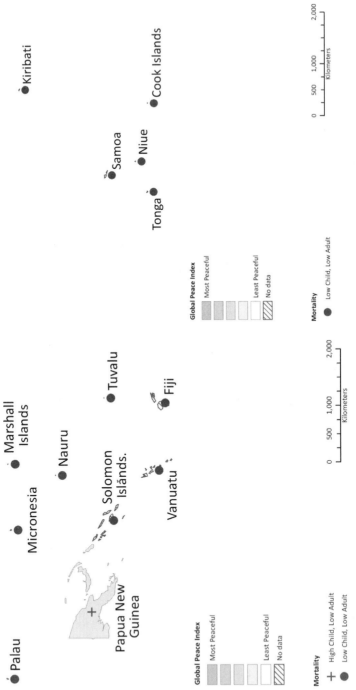

OFFICIAL LANGUAGE(S)

28 official languages, including:

- Fiji, Kiribati, Marshall Islands, Micronesia, Nauru, Palau, Papua New Guinea, Samoa, Solomon Islands, Tonga, Tuvalu, Vanuatu = English
- Vanuatu = French
- Timor-Leste = Portuguese
- Fiji = Hindi

"I first began visiting Papua New Guinea on holiday at Easter 2003. Following this visit, I contacted the Dean of the Medical and Health Sciences Faculty at the University of Papua New Guinea. This led to a health promotion initiative with members of the Kewapi language group who originate from the Southern Highlands and who live in a settlement in Post Moresbey. The settlement is behind Jackson's international airport and is 1 hour's flight away from Cairns in Australia, yet 47 people share one stand pipe for water and there is no electricity or other source of power other than scavenged wood-burning fires.

Papua New Guinea has an equatorial climate mediated by the mountainous terrain of the country. The mountainous terrain interspersed with dense jungle, vast rivers and poor transport infrastructure make it difficult for remote communities to access even basic services such as health and education. This leads many people from the Highlands region to gravitate to Port Moresby.

The peoples of Papua New Guinea speak over 800 indigenous languages. These language groups result from the social isolation due to the difficult terrain. Each attests separate traditions and cultures. People can identify closely with a tight family grouping. This occurs despite lack of access to telecommunication, information technology and very poor transport infrastructure.

I have really enjoyed working with these communities and particularly one of the elders, Dr Willie Ako. He has acted as in-country advisor and facilitator to the project. This involved translation and interpretation to represent the views of his community. He has great enthusiasm and commitment, and has allowed me great insight into this culture."

Dr Jane Fitzpatrick, senior lecturer, Adult Nursing School, University of the West of England

Find out more

- WHO regional office website: *http://www.wpro.who.int*

Europe

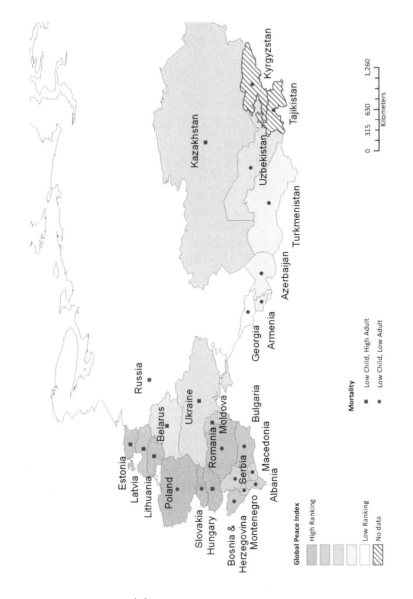

Mortality
- ■ Low Child, High Adult
- ● Low Child, Low Adult

Global Peace Index

High Ranking

Low Ranking

No data

OFFICIAL LANGUAGE(S)

National languages, but Russian spoken widely in former USSR states

"I have researched and taught in Ukraine for the last 30 years and now hold a UNESCO Chair there. I was invited initially by a team of scientists working in low-temperature biology.

I found that the team was producing good results, but was totally isolated. They were incredibly welcoming, as they were desperate for outside contact. The central control structure was suffocating, and there was no understanding of the need for long-term investment in scientific institutions. Due to the state paranoia, people kept their head down and avoided sticking their neck out on issues. It wasn't uncommon for esteemed professors to be chucked out of their positions because they had upset a party member, whatever the quality of their science.

Teaching was difficult as the students were very well versed in theory, but were very respectful of age and wouldn't argue with me! Socialising with colleagues was tricky at first. You really do have to be able to hold your alcohol, and it was and to a degree still is a very male-dominated society.

Everything collapsed after 1989, including science and health. I knew professional colleagues who were begging on the street. Things are improving gradually now, and there's much more openness."

Professor of surgical science, Ukraine

Find out more

- WHO regional office website: *http://www.euro.who.int*

REFERENCES

Department for International Development (2007). *Preventing Violent Conflict (Policy Paper)*. London: DFID.

Fitzpatrick J, Ako WY (2007). Empowering the initiation of a prevention strategy to combat malaria in Papua New Guinea. *Rural and Remote Health* 7: 693.

Global Peace Index. http://www.visionofhumanity.org/.

Hill P, Farooq G, Claudio F (2010). Conflict in least-developed countries: challenging the Millennium Development Goals. *World Health Organization Bulletin* 88(8):561–640.

Humanitarian Policy Group (2009). *Delivering Aid in Insecure Environments: Briefing Paper 34*. London: Overseas Development Institute.

Lewis MP (ed) (2009). *Ethnologue: Languages of the World*, 16th edition. Dallas: SIL International.

Merlin (2010). *A Grave New World* (Merlin Campaign Paper). London: Merlin.

Sheik M, Gutierrez MI, Bolton P, Spiegel P, Thieren M, Burnham G (2000). Deaths among humanitarian workers. *British Medical Journal* 321:166, doi: 10.1136/bmj.321.7254.166.

World Health Organization (2003). *World Health Report: Shaping the Future*. Geneva, WHO.

World Health Organization (2006). *World Health Report: Working Together for Health*. Geneva, WHO.

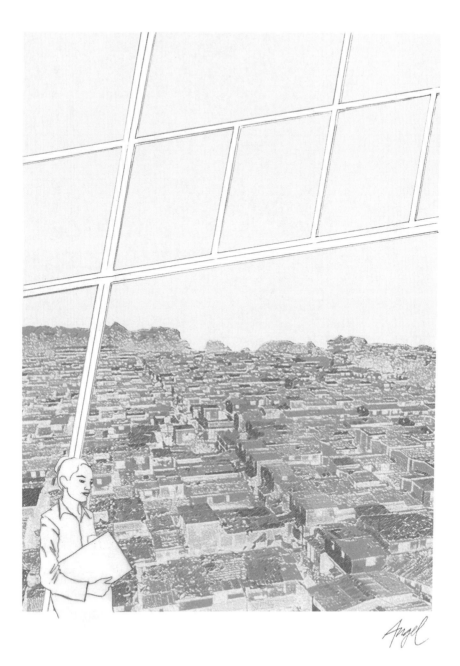

CHAPTER 7

Planning your placement

Chapter 5 introduced you to the types of work available and Chapter 6 gave an overview of where you could work. Having read these chapters you should have a clearer idea of your preferences. So how can you now find a suitable placement?

You have several options when planning your time overseas. One is to go through an organisation that recruits UK health professionals for international placements. This might be in a voluntary or paid capacity. Or you could arrange a placement directly with a hospital or local organisation, by either responding to an advertised vacancy or approaching them directly. Alternatively you could pay an organisation to arrange a tailor-made placement for you. Finally, you could sign up to a register that deploys health workers to organisations as and when needed.

This chapter will help guide you towards the right option for you. The first section takes you through the process of deciding whether to go with an established organisation; and, if not, how you can arrange your own placement. The second part is a directory of some of the most common organisations that recruit health professionals for international work.

First steps

Draw up your wish-list

In order to refine your search, it is useful to jot down your priorities. Consider the questions in Table 7.1.

Table 7.1 Drawing up your wish-list

Criteria	Preferences
Duration: how long do you want to work for?	Do you want to take time out from an NHS career to get involved in international work, turn it into a full-time job, or are you restricted to shorter placements which are compatible with an NHS career?
Geographical area: where do you want to be?	Think about languages, personal interests, access, safety, urban or rural preference (also consider where the local need for your skills is the greatest), schooling (if you have children) and social opportunities
Type of work: what do you want to do?	Humanitarian or development work? Clinical, teaching, research, project management?
Contract type: paid or voluntary?	Can you afford to cover all of your own costs, or do these need to be covered? Do you want to get a salary on top of this?
What you can offer?	What skills and experience do you have?
What do you want to get out of it?	What are your reasons for doing it? What do you hope to learn from the experience?

For **electives**, you will definitely be a volunteer with a fixed duration, but consider some other aspects:

- **Do you go with friends or on your own?** Friends provide safety in numbers and are great travelling companions, but you may have a more immersive experience by yourself.
- **Travel opportunities.** Most students combine electives with a great holiday. Factor this in to your location—can you travel overland anywhere or plan a stopover?
- Don't just feel **restricted to hospitals or clinics**. Could you work in a refugee camp or a research centre? Again, think about what experience you want to get out of it and mould this opportunity to your future career interests.

Organisational search

There are several advantages of working through an established organisation, so it is worth researching this option in detail before embarking on the route of organising your own placement. Some of the benefits of going with an organisation are that they are likely to:

- Recruit you for a **specific position** based on local need
- Try to ensure that you have the **appropriate skills** for the post

- Provide **support** from the time you are recruited—in the form of pre-departure preparation and briefings—all the way through to your return and beyond
- Support your posting overseas **financially**, whether it is a full salary, local salary or just travel and subsistence costs (although some, such as those organising electives and 'tasters', may expect you to pay for your placement; see below)

If you work overseas with a reputable organisation, colleagues and managers may recognise and support you to a greater extent as they are more likely to be familiar with the organisation's work and reputation. Note that if you want to work in humanitarian emergencies, going through a reputed organisation is essential (see Chapter 8).

If you do match one or several organisations' criteria, and they match yours, it is advisable to follow this route. Start applying early as the time between the application process, selection and going overseas can be between 3 and 12 months, depending on the organisation. With some organisations you apply for a specific vacancy, while others maintain your CV on a database and contact you when they require someone with your skills.

Organisational principles

Do be aware that each organisation has founding principles which influence the way in which they work.

For example, some FBOs require those who work with them to share their religious standpoints, and these may be reflected in their daily work. Other organisations oppose certain faith teachings. For example, some organisations working in reproductive health have condemned the Catholic Church's stance on contraception. And whilst most organisations advocate on behalf of vulnerable populations, some have engaged politically whilst others guard their neutrality zealously.

When selecting your organisation, remember that you will be an ambassador for them and will need to promote their principles during your work.

Organising your own placements

What if you can't find an international organisation to suit your needs and you decide to organise your own placement directly?

You could look at websites that post vacancies or job listings for health professionals overseas. If you follow this route, you can be more sure that you are responding to local demand. The directory at the end of this chapter lists some of these websites.

If you decide instead to contact a hospital or organisation directly, you'll probably need to put in more work at the research, planning and preparation stages. How can you find a placement that suits your skills and experience?

- **Use your contacts.** Everyone knows someone who has done work overseas. See if your hospital or community has any Health Links (see Chapter 4) or ongoing collaborations overseas.

- Contact your reciprocal **professional council** (or the ministry of health if it doesn't exist) within the country you want to work in. Their embassy or high commission in the UK might also be able to help. They may have established initiatives to recruit people in the health sector and can refer you on to relevant people.
- **International professional associations** can often help with contact details of local associations; for example, the International Council of Nurses (http://www.icn.ch), the Commonwealth Nurses Federation (http://www.commonwealthnurses.org) and the International Confederation of Midwives (http://www.internationalmidwives.org).
- Go through the **directory** at the end of this chapter; it lists organisations that can organise a placement for you (under the 'You Pay' section) and websites with job listings.
- If you are interested in working in a **private hospital** contact the HR department directly. Some will also have websites that advertise their vacancies.
- If all else fails, you can research institutions and organisations that are working in your area of interest by a **Google or PubMed search**. Type in your interests, for example 'mental health, Nepal'. This may reveal organisations and research teams working in this area, which you can then go on to contact.

Be prepared to start early and chase up. Emails and letters often go unanswered, so try to telephone where you can and follow up in writing. International Reply Coupons can be bought from the Post Office which your contact can exchange for stamps to return your letter, although these days even the remotest parts of the world are connected to e-mail. Track down individuals' names if at all possible—a personal approach goes a long way. Keep copies of all correspondence and take these with you.

Elective advice

All the tips above are relevant for electives, but also remember:

- Medical schools usually keep **elective reports** submitted by previous students. Do look at the ones in your preferred locations, as they're a good way to predict whether you will get the experiences you want out of it.
- The *Student BMJ* used to publish elective reports. These can be accessed http://archive.student.bmj.com/topics/travel/electives_and_exchange_programs.php
- *The Medic's Guide to Work and Electives Around the World* (see Appendix 2) and the associated website *http://www.medicstravel.org* has contact details for medical schools and hospitals around the world.

- By organising your own placement you will have a relatively free rein on where you go and what type of work you engage in. But try to ensure that it is based on local demands and fits in with the NHS Framework on International Development (see Chapter 13), by checking that:
  - The role you will be doing is based on local priorities (locally owned)
  - You will be working toward their goals rather than your own ideas of what you should be doing (aligned)
  - It is harmonised with other initiatives rather than duplicating efforts. For example, some hospitals may be saturated with international volunteers, while others receive little support
  - Due consideration has been given to what will happen after you leave— will you be leaving a gap or will local people be trained to continue your work (sustainable)?

Top tip

Rather than sending out your CV to a local organisation, a better starting point is to ask them what the needs of their organisation are, i.e. what vacancies they currently have and who they would be interested in recruiting as a volunteer. That way you can ensure a better match between your skills and the organisation.

Funding a placement

If you are not receiving a salary or volunteer stipend, you will probably be looking to raise money towards your placement, unless you want to use your savings. Due to the emotive nature of this work and high status of health professionals, raising funds can be very successful. Here are some tips for your appeal:

- Set up a fundraising page. Possible websites include Virgin Money Giving (uk.virginmoneygiving.com/giving/) and Mosaic Appeals (http://www.mosaicappeals.com/). JustGiving (http://www.justgiving.com) only sets up fundraising pages for registered charities.
- The Directory of Social Change (http://www.dsc.org.uk) lists grant-making bodies by typical areas of funding and target countries. For example, you could search for 'medical training' in 'South East Asia' or 'Cambodia'. See if your institution's library has a copy as you have to pay for online access.
- Ask if your employer will support your fundraising in some way, e.g. including your appeal in internal newsletters or a link on the hospital website.
- Use a variety of fundraising events, from the stalwart cake sale to the wacky sporting challenge. See http://www.better-fundraising-ideas.com for inspiration.

- Most medical schools have a pot of funding reserved for electives. Find out early what the selection criteria are for funding, and market your elective accordingly.
- Check if your professional association offers any grants. For example, the Royal College of Midwives offers a Student Travel Award each year.
- The British Medical and Dental Students Trust and other grant-making bodies offer specific bursaries for clinical electives. However, apply early as it's often first come, first served. See *http://www.money4medstudents.org* for further grants (useful for all professions).
- Work a research project into your elective. This way, you will be eligible for many more grants than for a clinical placement alone. For example, the Royal Society of Medicine offers the Brooke Bursary to electives involving a public health or epidemiology project.
- Write an article on your experiences. For example, the Anglo-French Medical Society offers a small payment for any report on an elective in a Francophone country, and the *RCM Midwives Journal* pays for articles too.
- Your old schools and local Rotary Club are good targets. Send a begging letter.
- Be aware that most institutions will charge you a fee for hosting your elective. This can be nominal in many countries, but factor it into your overall costs.

Accepting a placement

Whether you have been offered several placements or just the one, you will need to evaluate the position carefully before accepting it.

It is vital that you only accept a job for which you have the right competencies. Expectations differ between countries; for example, in many low-income countries very junior doctors are expected to provide the general surgical service in rural hospitals, whereas UK trainees at the same level will have had much less theatre time. Don't assume that because an organisation has offered you a post, it has fully evaluated your suitability. It may be more influenced by the urgency of filling the post. Only you can decide if you have the skills for the job.

Read Chapter 11 to help you understand the conditions under which you may be working overseas and to ask the right questions about the post.

- Find out exactly what will be expected of you. Evaluate this against your competencies.
- Ask what support and supervision there will be, especially for junior doctors and those on elective.
- If doing clinical work, ask to be put in contact with a colleague to find out about his/her case-mix.
- If your role will have a strong element of capacity building, find out who you will be training. How big is the team and what qualifications do they have?

If working for a humanitarian/emergency organisation, check that:

- It is well established, irrespective of its size (i.e. it is not an organisation that has been set up immediately after a disaster)
- It adheres to an internationally recognised code of conduct for humanitarian organisations, e.g. the code of conduct of the International Red Cross and Red Crescent Movement, or the People in Aid Code of Good Practice (see Chapter 11 for further information)
- You are happy with their risk assessment and security procedures, care for staff (such as R&R breaks) and pre-departure briefings and preparation

Organisations you could work with

This next section looks at organisations that recruit health professionals for international placements. The first part features ten major organisations in detail and then goes on to provide a summary of other categories: organisations where you pay, where they pay and job-listing websites.

While we have listed many of the major organisations working in this field, the lists are not comprehensive and should be complemented by your own research. We have prioritised UK-based international organisations, but have on occasion mentioned others.

The focus of the listed organisations is health and/or humanitarian assistance. Of course, other options do exist in other sectors, such as water and sanitation, but these are beyond the scope of this chapter.

Doctors of the World (DOW)

DOW is an international humanitarian organisation providing medical care and advice to vulnerable people in the UK and overseas. Their international projects focus on emergency response efforts, rehabilitation and reconstruction, and long-term, sustainable healthcare development. Key areas are mother and child health, HIV/AIDS, primary healthcare, street children, climate change and migration.

WHO THEY RECRUIT

Doctors (medical coordinators), surgical staff, obstetricians, psychiatrists, nurses, midwives, logisticians, financial administrators, general coordinators and field coordinators (a medical background is advantageous but not essential for these positions).

RECRUITMENT PROCESS

Initially, send your CV with a brief covering letter to the HR director. This will be followed by a face-to-face interview at the UK office and then a phone interview with headquarters in Paris. If successful you will be asked to go to Paris for a face-to-face. If successful, pre-departure training and briefings also take place in Paris.

"From the start of my career as a midwife I wanted to work abroad. In preparation I took the courses to better prepare me: a Diploma in Tropical Nursing, Examination of the Newborn and Advanced Life support in Obstetrics.

I met DOW at a careers fair and I liked their emphasis on training local staff. I was offered a 6-month placement in the remote Somali region of Ethiopia as a Traditional Birth Attendant (TBA) Trainer. In the absence of other medical facilities, training TBAs is an important means to improve maternal health. My assignment was to facilitate training and monitor TBAs activities in the region. The courses were designed to aid the identification of high-risk pregnancies and potential complications in labour.

My overall first impression, aside from the desert heat and dust, was that there was a lot of work to be done, which was exciting. The team (all local with one expatriate) were really welcoming. I spent the first month planning and then started teaching. I really enjoyed the interaction with the local population, but teaching was challenging given the low levels of education. I made it interactive: using pictures, role plays and fake blood. I got the rather reserved TBAs to laugh with my ridiculous acting and participate with role plays and storytelling.

Living conditions were adequate, but fresh fruit and vegetables were limited so we mainly lived off pasta. The Somali region is a conflict zone and there was a risk of kidnapping. DOW has strict security rules which are continually updated, so I felt well prepared for the situation.

The work did require the ability to adapt quickly to changing situations. Working in culturally diverse London prepared me well. But it is important to be under no illusion that you will be saving the world. I remain hopeful that some of the work we do can make changes in people's lives and encourages community action.

Once back I immediately started temporary work at my old hospital and then a promotion in a new hospital. I felt an increased confidence—in terms of gaining teaching and basic managerial skills."

Anne Fuller, Midwife, Ethiopia, March to October 2009

At a glance

Voluntary	−£	£ =0	£	££	*Paid*
Emergency context					*Development context*
Short term					*Long term*
Number of people recruited in 2010	300		*Top 5 countries of operation in 2010*		Ethiopia, Haiti, Liberia, Pakistan, Sudan

Advantages	• Make a real difference in emergency situations and in the longer term • Cooperate with local communities and authorities in order to make sustainable improvements to existing structures • Being part of DOW's advocacy efforts gives people a voice and helps volunteers to develop their resourcefulness • Work with local staff so that you can learn from them and they can learn from you.
Disadvantages	• Must have previous experience • Previous experience of working in the field is desirable; however, more importantly you should have professional qualifications and have worked in the UK in a professional capacity • Living and working in potentially unstable countries
Essential criteria for recruitment	• Minimum 2 years of post-qualification experience • Relevant professional and field experience are required • Availability at short notice • Adaptable and able to work in a team • Ability to train others and pass on skills
Desirable criteria	• Qualification in tropical medicine • Travel or work experience in LMIC • Foreign language skills

Length of placements	• Emergencies: a few weeks to 3 months
	• Post-crisis projects: 4–7 months (with the possibility of renewal)
	• Long-term development projects: 9–12 months (with the possibility of renewal)
Costs covered	• Transport from home to the assignment
	• Accommodation during the assignment
	• £260 per month for living and subsistence costs (or more depending on the country and type of programme)
	• Monthly allowance of £700 (£800 for coordinators; around £1,740 for salaried posts)
	• Medical and other insurance
Find out more	DOW runs recruitment days and careers fairs, advertised on the website or contact the HR director. *http://www.doctorsoftheworld.org.uk*, 14 Heron Quays, London E14 4JB. Tel: +44 (0)20 7515 7534

Mercy Ships

Mercy Ships is an international Christian charity that provides free medical care, relief aid, community assistance and long-term sustainable development in the poorest countries in the world. It runs the world's largest charity hospital ship—the *Africa Mercy*—and over the last 30 years has worked in over 70 countries. It runs medical and dental clinics, performs surgery and also gets involved in community development projects that focus on water and sanitation, education, etc.

WHO THEY RECRUIT

Doctors (anaesthetists and specialists in maxillofacial/ENT, urogynaecology (vesico-vaginal fistulae), ophthalmic, orthopaedics, general surgery, plastic surgery (burns, ear reconstruction, tendon transfer for leprosy), dentists, opticians, registered nurses, community health educators, mental health and palliative care, community development personnel (engineers, builders, agriculturalists), cooks, cleaners, teachers, marine staff (officers, engineers, mechanics, pursers, health and safety, deck hands).

RECRUITMENT PROCESS

Short-term and long-term posts are available and advertised on the website, or the Stevenage office can be contacted directly for more information.

"As a Christian, I always wanted to use my skills to help others, but it took many years to prepare for the volunteering I do now. I am both a scrub nurse and an anaesthetic nurse so I am flexible which is really useful on the ship.

A colleague who had volunteered with Mercy Ships suggested I would enjoy it. As an operating theatre nurse the ship offers me the best place to use my skills when I can only offer a few weeks of service. I work in the Operating Theatre Department, but in Benin I was also privileged to teach local nurses.

The work is so different from home. The patients are more challenging as their diseases are far more advanced and they often arrive malnourished because of the nature of their disease. No two days are the same. On board you feel you belong to a special community and everyone is there to do their best for the patients. One day I counted 12 nationalities of volunteers in the theatre, so there are huge opportunities to learn from each other.

Pre-departure preparation was thorough and I was given the chance to 'buddy' with someone before I went—it's a great system.

The sense of being able to use one's skills in a place where patients are so appreciative cannot be measured. You have to be prepared for working in different ways and also for the fact that the experience will change you. I found it hard to settle back into life at home and 'normal' work, so make sure you discuss things with your close family as the person who left will not be the same person who returns.

I still serve as a short-term volunteer and in between am a bank nurse in the UK. To help with my work on board the ship, I have gained a Diploma in Community Eye Health from LSHTM and have undergone a 1-month course in Texas, offered by the charity.

Alison Herbert, theatre nurse, Togo/Benin/Liberia/Sierra Leone

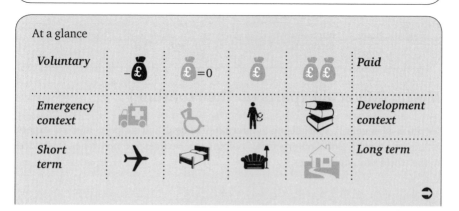

At a glance					
Voluntary	-£	£=0	£	££	*Paid*
Emergency context					*Development context*
Short term					*Long term*

Number of people recruited from the UK in 2010	148	*Top 5 countries of operation in 2010*	Togo and South Africa. The ships only visit one or two countries a year

Advantages	• Opportunity to work in state-of-the-art hospital environment and learn from international colleagues • Short term, so little disruption to career • Sometimes able to accommodate couples if housing allows and both have a role on the ship
Disadvantages	• No costs are covered
Essential criteria for recruitment	• Requires at least 2 years of post-graduate experience before volunteering for most clinical positions in the hospital • Must hold an active licence in good standing in your home nation
Desirable criteria	• Willingness to volunteer for more than 3 months. Experience working/living in confined spaces
Length of placements	• A minimum commitment is specified for each position, based on the orientation required and need for consistency. While it is easier for a member of the surgical team to come for only 2 weeks, ward nurses require a more extensive orientation and therefore come for a minimum of 2 months.
Costs covered	• Volunteers need to cover/raise their own costs to cover crew fees and flights. Individuals must cover their own insurance costs as well.
Find out more	*http://www.mercyships.org.uk*. The Lighthouse, 12 Meadway Court, Stevenage SG1 2EF. Tel: +44 (0)1438 727800

Merlin (Medical Experts on the Frontline)

Merlin is a UK charity specialising in international health. It supports medical experts on the frontline of global emergencies, helping to save lives and revive health services in the world's toughest places.

WHO THEY RECRUIT

Surgeons, nurses, midwives, public health doctors/nurses, primary health coordinators, nutritionists, epidemiologists, country health directors, reproductive health offiers.

RECRUITMENT PROCESS

Apply to advertisements for specific jobs posted on Merlin's website. You will have a first and second telephone interview. Some posts also require written tests. If selected you will have an induction at the head office in London.

"I wanted more of a challenge in my job, so I chose to work overseas with Merlin. They are the only British humanitarian organisation working (exclusively) in health and I like their philosophy of strengthening healthcare systems. But the work can be addictive. Since starting with Merlin I have had placements in countries as diverse as Siberia, Chechnya, Tajikistan, Afghanistan, the West Bank, Albania, Kosovo, Darfur and the Philippines. I was awarded an MBE for my work with Merlin in 2001.

My favourite experience was training female community health workers in Afghanistan. I had to travel to very remote mountainous areas by donkey and persuade the elders to let them be trained. At first there was reluctance as they said their women were ignorant, but I managed to convince them that illiteracy was no barrier to learning. Using different training methodologies they overcame their shyness and now they are delivering effective healthcare to the women and children in their communities.

We also started the first residential School for Rural Midwives in Takhar, Afghanistan. Following strict rules to ensure the school was culturally acceptable, I was there to see the first cohort of 22 students graduate.

More recently I took up a post on an island in the Philippines restoring health services after floods and typhoon Ondoy. Living and working with the affected people gives a better understanding of their problems and working together to find solutions.

I love the diversity of the work and enjoy living and working in another culture. It has given me access into people's lives that would never be possible as a tourist. There is a great range of work possibilities and a chance to really make a difference and a good way to share your skills."

Valerie Powell, nurse and midwife

Voluntary					Paid
	$-£$	$£=0$	$£$	$££$	
Emergency context					Development context
Short term					Long term

Number of people recruited from the UK in 2010	20	Top 5 countries of operation in 2010	Democratic Republic of Congo, Liberia, North Sudan and South Sudan, Pakistan, Haiti

Advantages	• Young, dynamic and flexible organisation • Many opportunities for individuals to get actively involved in organisational and programme development. We are a learning organisation, evaluating our programmes and using this learning to constantly inform and enhance the effectiveness of our work • Programmes in a wide variety of countries and operating contexts give the opportunity for individuals to develop skills and experience at a variety of levels and in a variety of settings
Disadvantages	• Work in extremely challenging, often highly insecure countries, where the general and health infrastructure and capacity are extremely weak and resource poor • Teams often live in communal houses and work in remote environments, with very limited ability to maintain regular communication with friends and family
Essential criteria for recruitment	• Qualified doctor or nurse with extensive post-qualification experience, some of which should be international in relief context • Qualification in tropical medicine and/or public health • Information analysis, report writing and analytical skills

	• Demonstrated analytical and conceptual skills to plan projects, timetable agreed activities and oversee staff activities • Good knowledge and experience of running primary healthcare projects, e.g. vaccination campaigns, response to disease outbreak, mobile clinics in LMIC • Competence in epidemiological analysis and knowledge of data collection methods and data analysis skills
Desirable criteria	• Masters in Public Health • Diploma in Tropical Medicine and Hygiene • Strong written and spoken French
Length of placements	• Between 6 months and 2 years
Costs covered	• Competitive salary range (depending on location and accommodation) • Health and personal possessions insurance • Transport to and from project location • Vaccinations and malaria prophylaxis • Excess luggage allowance • Additional flight home after 12 months' service • Minimum 24 days' annual leave and public holidays • Rest and relaxation breaks from hardship locations
Find out more	All vacancies are advertised on the website and on ReliefWeb. Merlin also attends recruitment days at LSHTM and LSTM *http://www.merlin.org.uk*. 12th Floor, 207 Old Street, London, EC1V 9NR. Tel: +44 (0)20 7014 1600

Médecins Sans Frontières (MSF)

MSF is an independent humanitarian medical aid organisation. It is committed to providing medical aid where it is most needed, regardless of race, religion, politics and gender. It also raises awareness of the plight of the people it helps.

WHO THEY RECRUIT

Doctors (including anaesthetists and surgeons), nurses, midwives, epidemiologists, mental health specialists, biomedical scientists, non-medical professionals (logistics, finance, water and sanitation, administration, HR).

RECRUITMENT PROCESS

Apply online using the application form. If your interview screening is positive, you will be invited for interview. Post-interview checks include two professional references, criminal record bureau and medical registration. If the interview outcome is positive, you will undergo a matching process which is based on the needs of the field and the candidate's availability, skills and experience. Pre-departure preparation course and comprehensive briefings follow a confirmed position.

"After graduating in 2002, I worked as an intensive care nurse at in the UK. But I let my passion for travel take me to Costa Rica, Nicaragua and finally to MSF.

The next thing I knew, I was on my way to South Sudan for a 9-month placement. I spent about half my time working as an outreach nurse in rural communities, and the other half in a hospital in-patient feeding facility as a base nurse.

The work was definitely challenging, and so much different than anything I'd done before. I would see thousands of patients a month, so I hardly had time to think. Logistics made it difficult to diagnose and provide care for patients: simple things like patient histories are non-existent. Because the level of education is so low, patients don't know about common health problems like pneumonia, and explaining basic things like how to take tablets could be really difficult. Combined with the language barrier, the situation was a nightmare sometimes.

Seeing people suffering was also very hard. Some patients were walking for days to get to healthcare and would arrive in a terrible state. Watching children dying of malnutrition doesn't get any easier with time. The situation was a bit desperate, and it definitely took its toll.

There were positive things about the experience, though. There's nothing better than seeing a bouncing, lively child discharged home where previously they were unable to stand. Also, because the teams live in such close quarters, you make friends for life.

I've been on two more missions since: one in Sudan and one in Papua New Guinea. Working with MSF has made me so much more appreciative of what we have here. The most frustrating thing since being back is hearing about people not getting their children vaccinated in the UK when it's freely available. Being out there puts a lot into perspective, and you have to be ready for it."

Stephen Flannagan, emergency nurse, South Sudan and Papua New Guinea

At a glance					
Voluntary	–£	£=0	£	££	Paid
Emergency context					Development context
Short term					Long term
Number of people recruited from the UK in 2009	200	Top 5 countries of operation in 2009			Sudan, Democratic Republic of the Congo, Somalia, Ethiopia, Niger

Advantages	• Development of medical experience and skills • Development of 'soft' skills: communication, team work, training and management • Opportunities for a long-term career with MSF including internal and external training
Disadvantages	• Being away from friends and family for long periods of time • Long working hours in challenging environments with fewer resources than are available in the UK
Essential criteria for recruitment	• Significant and relevant professional experience • Minimum of 3 months' travel or work experience in LMIC • Willingness to work in unstable areas; flexible and able to manage stress • Commitment to the aims and values of MSF • Management experience combined with the ability to train others and pass on knowledge and skills
Desirable criteria	• Foreign languages, particularly French, Arabic and Spanish • Prior experience of working overseas/insecure environments (for example, with international NGOs) • Tropical medicine experience

Length of placements	• 9–12 months, with the exception of surgeons and anaesthetists whose placements are usually between 6 weeks and 6 months
Costs covered	• Costs are covered including pre-mission training, flights, visas, vaccinations, pre-mission health checks, accommodation and daily living allowance • Other benefits are a comprehensive insurance package, 28 days annual leave pro rata, an optional pension, and learning and development opportunities. In addition a basic starting salary is paid of approximately £700/€978 per month
Find out more	*http://www.msf.org.uk* (or *http://www.msf.org* internationally). 67–74 Saffron Hill, London EC1N 8QX. Tel: +44 (0)207 404 6600

Operation Smile

Operation Smile is an international organisation that uses medical volunteers to make a difference to the lives of children born with cleft lips and palates. International projects typically involve a team of healthcare volunteers who travel to more than 50 countries to provide free reconstructive surgery for children over a 2-week period. Patients also receive ongoing aftercare for speech and dentistry. Every project is treated as a training opportunity to provide local volunteers with the skills needed to treat patients all year round.

WHO THEY RECRUIT

Plastic surgeons, anaesthetists, paediatricians, paediatric intensivists, nurses, dentists, biomedical technicians, speech therapists, child psychologists and play therapists.

RECRUITMENT PROCESS

Go online to download a medical project application. All medical experts are credentialed locally and internationally, which can take up to 3 months to process. Where necessary, candidates may be required to undertake further training before joining a medical project.

"I first volunteered with Operation Smile in 1995 when I went on a 2-week project to Colombia. The experience was so uplifting and rewarding that I have been on projects every year since. One of the advantages of Operation Smile is that the projects are generally for 2 weeks. This means I can volunteer every year with minimal disruption to my job or family. It has given me the opportunity to work in Colombia, the

➲

Philippines, the West Bank, Romania, China, Kenya, Ethiopia and India. It is fascinating to work alongside other doctors, nurses and healthcare workers in their own, often challenging, environment. It always makes me realise how lucky we are to have the NHS.

Operation Smile has very robust criteria for selection of volunteers. You have to have the correct qualifications and credentials to be able to be accepted. This does mean that when you take part in a project you are surrounded by like-minded suitably qualified professionals. One of the down sides is that many people who would like to volunteer do not fulfil the professional criteria. I have never felt professionally vulnerable during any programme as there is always support available, both in personnel and equipment.

A highlight during a project is having the opportunity to help train the local doctors and nurses. During a project we might operate on 200 children. I have always looked upon this as 200 training opportunities. When I went on my first project to Colombia, virtually all of the 40 strong team was from outside Colombia. Now Operation Smile Colombia is totally self sufficient. All of the surgeons, anaesthetists and nurses are now from Colombia. The project is a success when we are no longer needed.

At the end of the day there is nothing more satisfying than seeing a child who has had their life changed and a mother or father who will be forever grateful. A word of warning: once you have been on an Operation Smile project it becomes increasing difficult to say no. I'm still going after 15 years!"

Phil McDonald, consultant anaesthetist, 1995–2010

At a glance

Voluntary					*Paid*

Emergency context					*Development context*

Short term					*Long term*

Number of people recruited from the UK in 2010	91 (over 4,000 worldwide)	*Top 5 countries they worked in in 2010*	India, Vietnam, the Philippines, China, Colombia

Advantages	• An opportunity to work with an international team of medical experts
	• Short-term placements, so compatible with a UK career
	• Training is key to what Operation Smile does—for both local and international volunteers. Sustainability is at the forefront of the organisation's methodology
	• A life-changing experience
Disadvantages	• Paediatric experience essential
	• Long hours with heavy schedules
	• Flexibility needed
Essential criteria for recruitment	• Minimum 2 years of post-qualification experience
	• Relevant professional and field experience
	• Availability at short notice
	• Adaptable and able to work in a team
	• Ability to train others and pass on skills
Desirable criteria	• Travel or work experience in LMIC
	• Foreign language skills
Length of placements	• Project—2 weeks including travel
	• Post-operative—1 week
	• Care centre work—up to 2 months
Costs covered	• International transport
	• Accommodation during a project visit
	• All meals (nearly always)
	• Medical, travel and repatriation insurance
Find out more	*http://www.operationsmile.org.uk.* Email: volunteers@operationsmile. og.uk. 15 The Coda Centre, 189 Munster Road, London SW6 6AW. Tel: +44 (0)844 581 1110

Skillshare International

Skillshare works in partnership with people, local organisations and communities in Africa and Asia and helps to support their development. One way it does this is by placing international volunteers in those organisations. It recruits skilled professionals for placements in a range of sectors, but health programmes are common. Skillshare focuses firmly on the needs of its partner organisations.

WHO THEY RECRUIT

A diverse range of health professionals. There are some medical roles, but the placements are more likely to be in public health, policy or project management rather than in clinical work. They also work in other areas including engineering, business, education and finance.

RECRUITMENT PROCESS

The application form is online. You can respond to a specific advertisement or go in via the general recruitment stream. Short-listed candidates will be interviewed and the selected volunteer taken though referencing, police checks and medical checks. There is a pre-departure training course as well as in-country orientation.

"I did an elective in Madagascar and was impressed by the work and dedication of the overstretched doctors that I met. I wanted to go back and work in a LMIC.

After I gained some experience and post-graduate qualifications I was ready to do this. Before Skillshare, I worked in Mozambique for two and a half years with VSO. During this time I saw a number of foreign doctors on 1- or 2-year contracts arrive, struggle to learn Portuguese and leave as soon as they were working effectively. I came to the conclusion that the medical school needed some longer-term support, at least until the first graduates had gained experience and the post-graduate qualifications to come back and replace me.

Consequently I was looking for an organisation that was committed to supporting me and the medical school for a number of years. This is why I chose to work with Skillshare International for 3 years as a Medical Lecturer and GP at the Catholic University of Beira, Mozambique.

My day-to-day work involved facilitating medical and nursing students' learning in clinical skills through their problem-based learning curriculum. I worked with Faculty staff, including some of our graduates, to develop skills, learning resources and assessment methods. Due to a lack of personnel and the fast turnover of staff I had to work for long hours.

Planning and getting things done was sometimes a challenge as staff from different backgrounds each had their own ideas about when a deadline actually became urgent. This has lead to me becoming more patient and tolerant of different ways of working.

Skillshare International supported the cost of flights and medical insurance. They also worked in partnership with the Faculty to improve the availability of trained personnel by placing other development workers there.

Besides teaching me Portuguese, my work in Beira increased my interest in medical education and led me to begin study for a Masters in Medical Education by distance learning in 2009. Now that I am back in the UK I am continuing with this course and hoping to divide my time between General Practice and teaching medical students."

Dr Zoë Anne Walker, GP, Mozambique, May 2007 to May 2010

At a glance

Voluntary	$-£$	$£ = 0$	$£$	$££$	Paid
Emergency context					Development context
Short term					Long term

Number of people recruited from the UK in 2010	16	Top 5 countries they operated in in 2010	Swaziland, Lesotho, Kenya, Tanzania, India

Advantages	• The placements are assessed, structured and designed to create a lasting impact. Many development workers go on to paid work in Africa or Asia after their placement • It is a good opportunity to gain experience in advising governments, university lecturing or advocacy • Most development workers travel to placement unaccompanied; however, some placements are open to families and couples
Disadvantages	• A long time may pass between the application submission and the placement commencing. Police checks, visas and medical checks can take several months, so it is a good idea to apply well in advance
Essential criteria for recruitment	• For professionals: a degree and a minimum of 2–3 years post-qualification experience • For young volunteers and electives: a recommendation letter, strong commitment to social justice and international development, good student records
Desirable criteria	• Some experience of work or travel in an LMIC
Length of placements	• On average 18 months, but there are also short-term placements and opportunities for corporate sponsor volunteers, youth volunteers (18–25 years old), medical electives and online volunteering

Costs covered	• The costs are only covered if there is project, corporate or other private funding for it (flights, accommodation, medical insurance and a small allowance) • You are also asked to raise between £800 and £1,500 or the equivalent towards their work
Find out more	*http://www.skillshare.org* or *http://www.skillshare.ie*. 126 New Walk, Leicester LE1 7JA. Tel: +44 (0)116 254 1862. Fax: +44 (0)116 254 2614

British Red Cross (BRC)

BRC is an international humanitarian organisation which helps people in crisis, whoever and wherever they are. It is part of a global voluntary network, responding to conflicts, natural disasters and individual emergencies. It helps vulnerable people in the UK and abroad prepare for, withstand, and recover from emergencies in their own communities. BRC is a leading provider of delegates to the International Federation of Red Cross and Red Crescent Societies (IFRC), the International Committee of the Red Cross (ICRC) and to bilateral projects managed directly from London.

WHO THEY RECRUIT

Doctors (including surgeons and public health specialists), nurses, physiotherapists, nutritionists, prosthetists and logisticians. Also experts in water and sanitation, organisational development, relief, project/programme managers, disaster management, livelihood/food security, Arabic-speaking protection/detention, HR, communications, information and finance.

RECRUITMENT PROCESS

Complete an online application form available on the website. If your experience is in line with their positions in the field, you will be invited to attend a selection day at their London offices (panel interview and group exercises). If you are successful at selection day, references and a criminal record check will be obtained. If satisfactory, you will be placed on their overseas delegate register.

All subsequent offers of employment are subject to passing a medical assessment and attending a basic training course, which acts as an introduction to the Red Cross/ Red Crescent movement.

"I took my first job with the Red Cross in 1982 and so far I have done about 30 overseas missions with them. Now that I have built up a reputation with the Red Cross, I just have to phone them up and within a month they will have found something for me.

➲

ICRC sends me to the most disadvantaged and difficult places on the planet, for example Afghanistan, Sudan and the Congo.

Everywhere has its interest and challenges. The great reward for me is working in teams of young enthusiastic health workers to the obvious benefit of wounded people. Most of my colleagues on missions are, unlike me, working in the NHS and do an overseas mission with the Red Cross every few years.

The medical team on any mission tends to consist of five people, working in a local hospital with a team of 300 or more local staff. The heads of mission are excellent and team work is very important in these situations.

There is an element of training, as we are working side by side with local health workers. But when a war is going on we have to adopt a 'fire brigade' action. We are there to put the fire out. Words like sustainability are not terribly relevant in this context.

The Red Cross treats us well. I feel the pay is fair and correct; I am probably earning a third of what I would be in the UK, but tax free and with few expenses. A major concession for married couples is family reunion every 3 months consisting of 10 days leave back home, all costs covered. ICRC does try to place couples who are both working for it together.

As a generalist it would be difficult to return to a job in the UK in an increasingly specialist world. I would advise others to finish all relevant training prior to going, but then again by that time you might be married with three children as I was in 1974 and this could stop all thoughts of going. At least you should choose an adventurous spouse."

Kenneth Barrand, surgeon

At a glance

Voluntary					Paid
	−£	£=0	£	£ £	
Emergency context					Development context
Short term					Long term

Number of people recruited from the UK in 2010	45	Top 5 countries they operated in in 2010	Bangladesh, Haiti, India, Malaysia, Pakistan

Advantages	• All those who work with BRC, in whatever capacity, can expect to enter into a partnership which has at its core a clear commitment to providing the highest-quality service to vulnerable people. They have high expectations of their volunteers, staff and delegates, who in turn have high expectations of BRC
Disadvantages	• Together with the ICRC and IFRC, BRC works in conflict situations and are often the first agency to respond to natural disasters. This means that their international delegates may often live and work in challenging environments
Essential criteria for recruitment	• British nationals or UK residents • Must be adaptable, flexible and mature in judgment, should possess initiative, diplomacy, cultural sensitivity, and have the ability to live and work in a team, usually under arduous and sometimes dangerous conditions • Robust mental and physical health is essential • Must fully accept the Red Cross's Fundamental Principles and be prepared to acquire an understanding of the movement and its ideals
Desirable criteria	• Knowledge of foreign languages is always useful and encouraged, especially French, Arabic, Spanish or Russian
Length of placements	• Ranging from 1 month to 24 months

Costs covered	• Salary, ranging between £23,500 and £35,000
	• Return air travel
	• Cost of transport of personal effects
	• Medical and other insurance
	• War risk coverage
	• The ICRC undertakes to provide:
	  ▪ accommodation
	  ▪ local transport
	  ▪ variable mission allowance
	  ▪ mission allowance when applicable, in accordance with ICRC standards
	• Delegates are eligible for a paid home leave flight after 18 months of service. Excess baggage and unaccompanied freight allowances are also provided

- Delegates receive 6 weeks annual leave per year (3.5 days per calendar month). Delegates on contracts of 6 months or less are normally expected to take their annual leave after their mission
- Contracts of 12 months or more, security conditions permitting, are sometimes eligible for accompanied family status. Benefits include travel insurance, flights, child allowances and assistance with school fees

Find out more   The BRC holds 'selection days' to identify suitable candidates for the overseas delegate register and will otherwise advertise specific posts on the British Red Cross website. *http://www.redcross.org.uk*. 44 Moorfields, Moorgate, London EC2Y 9AL. Tel: 0844 8711111 from UK or + 44 2071 387900 from abroad. Email: recruitment@redcross.org.uk

RedR

RedR improves the effectiveness of disaster relief, helping save and rebuild the lives of people affected by natural disaster and conflict worldwide. It does this by delivering essential training and support to relief organisations and their staff and by providing skilled professionals to humanitarian programmes around the world.

WHO THEY RECRUIT

RedR does work on the frontline itself, but instead places experienced relief workers from its membership register in response to requests from frontline aid agencies. Currently, RedR has over 1,700 Members. RedR Members have extensive field experience in areas such as health, emergency shelter, water, logistics, sanitation and hygiene.

The health-related recruitment requests received are most likely to be for doctors, healthcare coordinators/managerial posts and nutritionists.

RECRUITMENT PROCESS

To apply for RedR membership, download and submit a completed application form from the website. If candidates are deemed suitable for potential RedR membership, they undergo a strict vetting process to ensure they have the right knowledge, skills and competencies to be deployed in an emergency situation. RedR checks professional references and conducts an intensive panel interview with experts in the candidate's area of specialisation.

This covers:

- Discussion of career history, particularly the nature of previous overseas assignments

- Assessment of competencies
- Consideration of managerial skills, from technical supervision to programme management
- Evaluation of personal qualities, including team-working skills, cross-cultural sensitivity and tolerance

"I have been working in the aid sector since the mid-1990s, where I worked with health care delivery and epidemiological assessments in several natural disasters (floods in Bangladesh, the Aceh tsunami and the earthquake soon after in Sumatra) as well as on other humanitarian aid missions.

Since starting out in the sector, I have undertaken a number of different RedR training courses and workshops—covering areas such as refugees, environmental health and needs assessment. The training that I have received from RedR has been indispensable in the field and they have also helped me professionally as I have been able to list them on my CV. In 2003, I became a RedR Member.

Following the Sichuan earthquake on 12 May 2008, I was part of a team of consultant surgeons and other emergency medical staff mobilised by RedR to fly out to China for the British FCO. I had several years' experience working in the public health sector in China and spoke Mandarin, so I was the natural choice to help facilitate the group.

The British team were asked to assist two hospitals. The first was in Mianyang Hospital, very close to the epicentre of the earthquake, where many local people were sleeping in tents, too afraid to stay in their homes. Here two Chinese trauma surgeons and a plastic surgeon were carrying out operations in the operating theatre, and the British accident and emergency doctor and nurse joined local colleagues in triage and stabilisation of new patients. Where needed, they would refer cases to the surgical team.

Complex trauma cases had been centralised in the second hospital. Here we consulted management and medical counterparts, and started carrying out operations. I joined the surgical team as photographer and auxiliary interpreter for two operations.

➲

It was a great experience to be part of this international cooperation and to have been able to help some of those injured in the earthquake. It was an interesting experience to see the Chinese disaster relief response close up: as a humanitarian aid professional I was impressed by the local rescue and relief efforts, as well as the Chinese ability to undertake damage limitation in view of imminent disasters through large-scale coordination."

Lucy Reynolds, Doctorate in Public Health (LSHTM), China 2008 earthquake

At a glance

Voluntary					*Paid*
Emergency context					*Development context*
Short term					*Long term*
Number of people recruited from the UK in 2010	RedR placed 17 Members	*Top 5 countries they operated in in 2010*		Haiti, Pakistan, Chile, Sudan, Democratic Republic of Congo	

Advantages	• They work with a range of organisations so you do not need to apply to each one individually
Disadvantages	• You need to have substantial previous experience to be accepted onto the register
Essential criteria for recruitment	• RedR Members all have some overseas humanitarian and/or development experience to be accepted onto the register, and most tend to be experienced aid workers
Desirable criteria	• Experience of disaster relief or post-conflict experience would be an advantage
Length of placements	• Placements vary according to the requests RedR receives, from permanent roles to short-term placements
Costs covered	• Dependent on recruiting organisation
Find out more	*http://www.redr.org.uk*. 250a Kennington Lane, London SW11 5RD. Tel: +44 (0)20 7840 6000. Email: info@redr.org.uk

United Nations Volunteers (UNV)

UNV programme is the United Nations organisation that promotes volunteerism to support peace and development worldwide. UNV directly mobilises more than 7,500 UN Volunteers every year nationally and internationally. More than 75% of UN Volunteers come from LMIC, and more than 30% volunteer within their own countries. Volunteers work across a range of sectors, including heath.

WHO THEY RECRUIT (HEALTH-RELATED)

UNV recruits health professionals from a broad range of specialisations both from clinical and non-clinical fields, for example, medical doctors, nurses, public health specialists and HIV/AIDS specialists.

RECRUITMENT PROCESS

Interested individuals should complete UNV's online registration form. When UNV receives a request for the services of a volunteer from a development partner, staff search the database for profiles that meet the requirements of the assignment.

Identified candidates are contacted and invited to express their interest and availability. After reviewing all responses received, a short-list of three to five profiles is submitted to the relevant partner requesting the services of a UN Volunteer. The requesting authorities make the final choice and select the candidate who best fulfils their needs and requirements, usually following an interview and/or in-depth assessment.

"It was in 2005 that I came across the UNV Limpopo Doctors programme, designed to assist the province's various health facilities through the provision of specialist doctors where there were critical shortages. I fondly remembered my first encounter with a Belgian volunteer I had worked with in a rural hospital in Ethiopia at an early stage of my career. So I too decided I would volunteer.

I still have a strong recollection of my arrival in Lebowakgomo Hospital in the rural township of Limpopo Province about 250 km from the South African administrative capital, Pretoria. I was working in a new hospital constructed in 1999 and run mostly by newly graduated doctors. I was given a wonderful welcome reception and a chance to introduce myself. I proudly said that I am an anaesthetist by profession and a UN Volunteer. The first question I was asked was whether a UNV assignment meant that I was stationed for a short time only? It was with this encounter that I started my primary role of advocating for volunteerism.

➲

I learnt about the unacceptable high rate of anaesthetic complications the hospital was facing, especially involving maternal anaesthetic complications. I could see the relief and appreciation my arrival had stirred among the young doctors.

The task of establishing and building up the anaesthesia unit kept me busy for the first months. The eagerness and dedication of the operation staff and doctors made it possible to quickly pass the first hurdle. We were able to markedly reduce the rate of anaesthetic referral cases to tertiary hospitals and in 2006–2007 we opened an Intensive Care Unit—a milestone in the history of our hospital.

In October 2008, I was awarded the best anaesthetist achievement award for outstanding performance and lasting contribution to innovation in the public service. This honour was not only in recognition of my personal contribution but also was an endorsement to all the UN Volunteers working in the province.

In my heart I will always be indebted to UNV for giving me this opportunity to apply my knowledge and experience for the benefit of society, to live and work among the South African people and learn their beautiful cultures. As it is beautifully expressed in local languages, I would like to end by saying, 'Re a Leboga' (thank you) to UNV."

Dr Abner Taye Kebede from Ethiopia, assistant professor and consultant anaesthesiologist in a university hospital, South Africa 2005–2008

At a glance

Voluntary				Paid
	–£	£=0	£	££
Emergency context	🚑	♿	🧑	📚	**Development context**
Short term	✈	🛏	🛋	🏠	**Long term**

Number of people recruited from the UK in 2010	60	Top 5 countries they operated in in 2010		48% of volunteers served in Sub-Saharan Africa

Advantages	• Receive the support of the UN network
	• Volunteers develop the capacities of the individuals and communities with whom they work, empowering them to find solutions to their challenges
	• Through this process, Volunteers can develop new skills, gain experience, build networks and motivate others to volunteer
Disadvantages	• UNV assignments are exciting and rewarding, but living conditions can be difficult or at times dangerous. Many Volunteers work in remote, isolated, duty stations and some operations are non-family assignments. Candidates are encouraged to refer to the UNV Conditions of Service before applying
Essential criteria for recruitment	• Commitment to the values of volunteerism
	• A university degree or higher technical diploma
	• Several years of relevant working experience
	• At least age 25 when taking up an assignment (there is no upper age limit)
	• Good working knowledge of at least one of the three UNV working languages: English, French or Spanish
Desirable criteria	• Previous volunteering experience
	• Experience abroad, especially in LMIC
Length of placements	• 6–12-month renewable contracts, with the expectation that the UN Volunteer will serve 1 year or more
Costs covered	• Settling-in grant calculated on duration of assignment, which is paid at beginning of assignment
	• Volunteer Living Allowance to cover basic living expenses, which is paid each month
	• Travel on appointment and at end of assignment as applicable
	• Life, health and permanent disability insurance
	• Annual leave
	• Resettlement allowance calculated based on duration of assignment, which is paid upon satisfactory completion of assignment
Find out more	*http://www.unvolunteers.org*. Postfach 260 111, D-53153 Bonn, Germany. Tel: +49-228-8152000. Email: information@unvolunteers.org

Voluntary Service Overseas (VSO)

VSO is an international development organisation that tackles poverty through volunteering. It mobilises skilled professionals to work with partner organisations in over 40 countries. VSO health volunteers train health staff, strengthen the management of health systems, empower communities to call for better healthcare, and support research for pro-poor policy.

WHO THEY RECRUIT

Doctors from a wide range of specialties (including surgery, medicine, paediatrics, obstetrics and gynaecology, general practice), nurses (community, general and mental health), midwives and health visitors, therapists (physiotherapists, occupational therapists, speech and language therapists), nutritionists and dieticians, health service managers, public health professionals, biomedical scientists.

RECRUITMENT PROCESS

Register and apply online, outlining your professional experience and availability. If you're available within 12 months, and VSO feels it's likely it will have a role for your skills and experience, you are invited to an assessment day and interview. If successful, VSO will discuss potential roles with you and your CV will be added to VSO's database. When a role is requested by a VSO partner, it searches the database and identifies a suitable individual. You are offered a role description and the time to research and consider it thoroughly. If the role is not for you, your details stay on the database until the next offer. Before travelling overseas you will undertake online learning and residential training courses.

"I travelled a lot in my 20s but felt it would be rewarding to stay in one place and really get to know a very different culture.

I chose VSO because I knew it was a large established organisation and had a history in this area; I also knew that with them I would be doing longer-term development work which would suit my strengths. Being a large organisation, I hoped VSO would have some choice of placements and a good number of other volunteers. I was concerned about being isolated (not a valid concern as it turned out) and therefore knew I wanted to be somewhere where I could get to a major town in a day.

I worked as a nurse/midwife consultant in a remote hospital in northern Cambodia and I was there for 21 months. Initially I only committed for a year, but as soon as I arrived I knew I could stay longer. We had 6 weeks' language training at the start, which was the envy of other volunteers. We were also given a lot of assistance in settling in to our placements and VSO kept in regular contact with us and was good at facilitating opportunities for us to meet other VSO volunteers.

⮑

I worked with the nursing and midwifery staff of the hospital to improve care. We had a small budget which went such a long way there. I was able to establish a nutrition project, improve care for high-risk pregnant women and initiate documentation for the nurses and midwives. I went back 2 years later and was delighted to see two of these projects still going.

The environment and the lack of infrastructure were big challenges. Much of the time it was very hot, we had intermittent electricity and the staff I was working with had many competing factors on their time. However, all these things made the achievements feel so much more rewarding.

VSO prepared us for coming home, but it was still quite a big shock to reintegrate back into your own society. I came back to work as a midwife in the NHS. I have taken three different roles in midwifery in the last four and half years. These have all been within the area of training and education. The overseas time taught me that small achievements are important and can add up to a very big whole."

Nikki Wales, midwife, Cambodia 2004–2005

At a glance

Voluntary				*Paid*
Emergency context				*Development context*
Short term				*Long term*
Number of people recruited from the UK in 2010	468	*Top 5 countries they operated in 2010*		Malawi, Cambodia, Cameroon, Ghana, Ethiopia

Advantages	• Work to strengthen existing health systems, within national health structures or civil society • Share skills with local colleagues, working together to bring about lasting improvements to health • Gain unique personal and professional development. Health professionals bring new perspectives back to the UK, along with deepened clinical, teaching and managerial skills
Disadvantages	• Most roles request a 1- to 2-year time commitment, in order to have a lasting impact • Health professionals generally need to be flexible about their destination. VSO's priority is that your skills are shared where they are most urgently needed • The process from applying to departing can take up to 12 months, depending on availability of roles and your personal circumstances, e.g. if you are volunteering as a couple
Essential criteria for recruitment	• Relevant professional qualifications and registration • At least 3–5 years' relevant professional experience • Some training, teaching or management experience • Flexibility and adaptability, commitment to learning, ability to work with others, cultural sensitivity, problem-solving ability
Desirable criteria	• Vary according to role: e.g. experience of working with HIV-positive patients
Length of placements	• 12–24 months; a small number of 3- to 6-month roles are available depending on professional background and level of experience
Costs covered	• Optional preparatory payment of £450 • Volunteering allowance (varies from country to country, according to cost of living, e.g. Cambodia £250 a month) • Return flight • Accommodation • Transportation, e.g. motorbike if needed • National Insurance contributions • Medical insurance, PEP and other medical kit • VSO small grants are available in-country for specific development projects with partner organisations
Find out more	'Meet VSO' events around the country, listed on *http://www.vso.org.uk/events*, and twice-yearly information days specifically for health professionals *http://www.vso.org.uk*. Carlton House, 27A Carlton Drive, Putney, London SW15 2BS. Tel: +44 (0)20 8780 7500. Email: enquiry@vso.org.uk

You pay

The following organisations arrange short- and medium-term placements in LMIC in exchange for a fee. If you are new to international health and want a guided experience, going through one of these organisations take a much of the hassle away from organising a placement yourself.

Some criteria you may want to use when choosing a fee-paying organisation are:

- Does it provide value for money?
- Does it provide pre-departure preparation such as briefings?
- Does it arrange visas and insurance?
- Does it provide support while you are there?
- Where does your fee go? Does it support the local community or is it for profit?
- Are they clearly responding to a need in-country?

Medical Student Electives (MSE)

Devised by the Charities Advisory Trust, MSE has teamed up with local NGOs in India and Rwanda to provide 4- or 5-week placements. They are planned and managed locally and provide an insight into rural and community health. Fifty to sixty people are placed each year. It costs around £1,250 and covers all accommodation and some transfers, but not air fares and insurance. Nursing electives can be arranged on an *ad hoc* basis and they accommodate specialties given advanced warning. Application is online and followed by a telephone interview. Placements are all year around. The money goes to support the organisations themselves and is not for profit. Their sister organisation also organises dental electives. They also welcome fully qualified doctors looking to experience medicine in India or Rwanda.

http://www.medicalstudentelectives.org
http://www.dentalstudentelectives.org

Work the World

This organisation is specifically aimed at organising electives for medics, nurses, midwives, dentists, radiographers and physiotherapists in Tanzania, Nepal, India, Sri Lanka, Argentina and Ghana. Their head office is in Brighton and they also have country offices in each of their destination countries which provide local support. Prices range from £940 for a 2-week placement to £1,640 for a 6-week placement. Cost includes detailed pre-departure preparation, placement organisation, privately rented accommodation, all food, and UK and overseas support. Work the World is a limited company, but it estimates that approximately 50–55% of the project fee goes directly to the overseas communities.

http://www.worktheworld.co.uk

Medics Travel

Originally set up to provide elective students with information on where to go, Medics Travel now also uses its network of contacts around the world to organise placements. For a fee of £85 they will link you with a placement that matches your criteria. You apply online, stating your preferred country of travel, dates and what you want to get out of it, and they will return up to 3 placements. They also produce *The Medic's Guide to Work and Electives Around the World*, a resource that includes information on hospitals, institutions and adventurous electives. Their website also has a jobs database.

http://www.medicstravel.co.uk

Projects Abroad

Within health, Projects Abroad organises volunteer and elective placements in medicine, physiotherapy, nursing and midwifery, dentistry, occupational therapy and speech therapy for all levels of experience. Placements are available in a wide range of countries in Africa, Asia and Latin America. Prices range from £1,195 for 2 weeks to £2,295 for 3 months and include all food and accommodation, transfers, travel and medical insurance, and support from local and UK staff. Costs do not include flight and visas.

http://www.projects-abroad.co.uk

They pay

Organisations that cover some or all of your costs while overseas, or offer a salary or generous living allowance, generally require you to be more senior within your profession and have some previous international experience. Many of the organisations listed below are registered NGOs or charities and generally receive funds for their activities from governments, grant-giving organisations and private donors. They often recruit for specific vacancies and undertake a rigorous selection process. Expect recruitment to be competitive. This list complements the detailed organisation descriptions in the second part of this chapter.

Catholic Relief Services (CRS)

CRS is the official international humanitarian agency of the Catholic community in the United States. CRS operates community health programmes in 26 countries serving approximately 3.5 million people. CRS focuses on providing healthcare for vulnerable groups in marginalised, unserved or underserved communities. The recruitment unit in Baltimore handles all employment applications.

http://www.crs.org

Doctors Worldwide (DWW)

DWW was established in 2000 to provide medical relief and aid to those who are in need without any access or means to basic medical care. It works in three key areas: (1) emergency relief, (2) extended medical relief post-crisis, and (3) rehabilitation, reconstruction and medical education. It recruits doctors, nurses, midwives, pharmacists, surgeons, mental health specialists and needs assessment specialists for short-term assignments. Whilst volunteers pay for their airfare, DWW provides local accommodation, transport and food.

http://www.doctorsworldwide.org

Global Medical Force (GMF)

GMF deploys expert medical professionals as 'clinical mentors' for 6- to 12-week field assignments. The main remit is the transfer of skills. They are looking for mentors from a wide variety of medical specialities including general medicine, primary care, paediatrics, obstetrics and gynaecology, HIV/AIDS, infectious diseases and emergency medicine. A minimum of 3 years' experience is required.

You need to complete an online application form and preparatory deployment workshops are held in New York, London, Sydney and South Africa. If selected, your airfare and local living expenses (hotel, accommodation and transportation) will be covered whilst on assignment.

http://www.globalmedicforce.org

HealthNet International

HealthNet International is a Dutch organisation which focuses on the structural rehabilitation of healthcare systems in fragile states. It recruits people with a professional background and solid experience in LMIC and in capacity building. They are looking for skills in the following areas: public health, disease control, health financing, health systems development, reproductive health, mental health, project management, finance and administration.

They offer both long-term contracts (1–3 years) and short-term contracts on a consultancy basis, depending on the nature of the assignment and donor funding.

http://www.hntpo.org/en

Medair

Medair recruits staff who are motivated by their Christian faith to care for people in need. Their headquarters are in Switzerland, but they have offices in London.

Medair's main focus is on primary healthcare, which includes both preventative and curative services.

All field candidates, new and experienced, must attend the week-long relief orientation course. Candidates pay the course fees and some travel costs. Remuneration for placements is calculated on years of relief work rather than on the level of experience or qualifications. New relief workers get most of their costs covered (food, lodging, medical insurance, vaccinations, local transport) and an allowance of US $100 per month. After 12 months this increases to between US $1,000 and US $3,500 per month. They run regular open evenings to provide information for prospective volunteers.

http://www.medair.org

ORBIS

ORBIS works towards eliminating avoidable blindness and bringing sight-saving care to LMIC. Medical volunteers are the backbone of ORBIS programmes, and placements last between 1 and 3 weeks. These specialists include ophthalmologists, orthoptists, biomedical engineers, anaesthetists and ophthalmic nurses. Volunteer ORBIS medical volunteers must be very highly experienced in ophthalmic eye care with a minimum of 5 years' practical experience at a consultant level for ophthalmologists and anaesthetists. Nurses must have 5 years' experience working in ophthalmic eye care. Refer to their website for details on how to volunteer. All costs incurred for volunteers are covered by ORBIS.

http://www.orbis.org.uk

Pharmacists Without Borders (PSF)

PSF was started in France and has a branch in Canada. Its goal is to establish optimal strategies for supplying essential medications and medical supplies where they are most needed. They take volunteers and paid staff.

http://www.psfcanada.org

International Medical Corps UK

This agency focuses on the provision of life-saving emergency health services, primary healthcare, public health and emergency nutrition. International Medical Corps recruits highly trained medical staff to add to their emergency response roster, which requires that volunteers be willing to deploy rapidly—usually within 72 hours—and for a duration of 2–8 weeks. Preference is given to those able to deploy for longer durations. In most instances, volunteers will be required to pay for their own flight but will receive a food allowance for each day spent in the field, shared housing and emergency medical evacuation insurance. They have offices in London, Los Angeles and Washington, DC.

http://www.internationalmedicalcorps.org.uk

Maldives International Volunteer Programme

The Maldivian High Commission in London and Friends of Maldives set up a partnership in 2008 to recruit health and education volunteers to the Maldives under the new democracy. They are actively recruiting UK health professionals, including doctors, nurses, social workers and drug rehabilitation workers to work alongside local health teams throughout the Maldivian islands. The main emphasis is on developing standards and sustainable systems through training, projects and improved governance. Placements are primarily 6–12 months but can be shorter under special circumstances.

Volunteers are given an allowance of US $700 per month and internal travel, lodging and energy bills are paid. The volunteers pay for their own flights to the Maldives.

http://www.friendsofmaldives.org http://www.maldiveshighcommission.org

Note that some other High Commissions may be involved in similar schemes and it is worth enquiring with them. They may at least be able to give you direct contacts to the Ministry of Health or health professionals within the country.

Career opportunities

If you are interested in making a full-time transition to international health work, there are many opportunities. Some of the organisations listed above recruit health professionals for full-time posts within their organisations; primarily in project management, advisory and policy roles. Alternatively many people take on assignment after assignment with an organisation they know and like. The following is a very selective list of other organisations that recruit for full-time posts. The final section gives an indication of where you might find other such job listings.

DFID

The UK's Department for International Development employs around 60 international health advisors for its overseas offices. All have 3–5 years' experience of work in LMIC health issues and a Masters degree in a relevant discipline (typically public health). They will be expected to work across a number of settings including fragile states. Once in post, they are expected to demonstrate understanding of broader development issues, particularly economics, aid effectiveness, governance and social development. Advisors require a deep understanding of health systems, the global health architecture and public health and population issues. A list of required technical competencies can be found on DFID's recruitment pages.

http://www.dfid.org

HLSP Healthcare Consultancy

HLSP provides health sector consultancy, programme management and policy advice to international agencies and national governments in LMIC. HLSP is supported by an in-house team of technical specialists and 8,000 external consultants offering a broad range of health sector skills, including health policy and planning, sector financing, governance, gender and capacity development.

Internationally, HLSP works in partnership with governments, bilateral and multilateral agencies, UN agencies, global health partnerships, foundations and private sector organisations. HLSP's expertise spans all aspects of health systems strengthening—from health policy and planning to sector financing, service delivery, governance and institutional development—and public health, including communicable diseases, maternal and neonatal health, and sexual and reproductive health.

http://www.hslp.org

Liverpool Associates of Tropical Health (LATH)

LATH has opportunities for short-term and long-term technical consultants. You can register online to be considered for consultancy posts. Minimum requirements include: a Masters level qualification or post-graduate professional qualification; at least 5 years' experience in the health sector; experience of short-term project work, for example, consultancy, research projects, or work as an external adviser; commitment to international health development; interest in pro-poor and gender-equitable approaches.

http://www.lath.com

Job listings

Christian Medical Fellowship (CMF)

CMF is not a sending agency but promotes and supports medical mission work by providing resources and information for doctors, nurses, therapists, dentists and students. Their website offers an extensive directory of FBOs and mission hospitals, and also advertises specific vacancies abroad. It runs the Developing Health course every year—a 2-week residential course for those preparing for work overseas (see Appendix 3).

http://www.cmf.org.uk

Mission Finder

This website lists work opportunities in Christian mission hospitals for health professionals and students.

http://www.missionfinder.org

International Medical Volunteers Association

This organisation provides information about volunteer opportunities and offers practical advice on how to find and choose compatible assignments. It works with a wide range of volunteers including doctors, dentists, nurses, therapists, hospital managers, public health specialists, physician assistants and students. It is based in the United States but has a comprehensive list of organisations that work in international health.

http://www.imva.org

Medical Missions

Medical Missions matches motivated healthcare professionals with organisations sponsoring medical missions. Organisations post vacancies on its website, which health workers can search. Its services are free for both medical volunteers and mission organisations.

http://www.medicalmissions.org/

ReliefWeb

ReliefWeb provides information and updates for those working in the emergency and development sectors and also has comprehensive job listings searchable by country and sector.

http://www.reliefweb.org

UN and WHO

This website lists all the internal and external vacancies available in different UN agencies. Look under WHO for health-specific ones.

http://www.unjobs.org

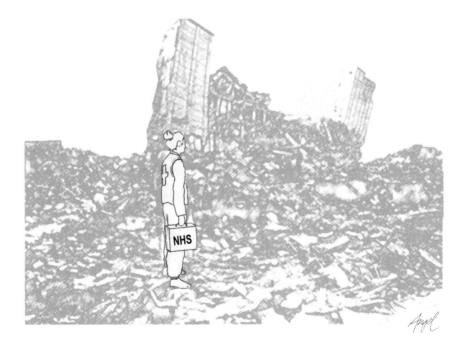

CHAPTER 8

Humanitarian relief

Most people are fortunate enough to experience a humanitarian crisis only on television: 'An earthquake has killed thousands and left many others homeless. . . . Fierce fighting has forced hundreds of thousands of people to flee . . . '. Crises like these, usually caused by conflict, famine or natural disasters, affect the lives of tens of millions of people around the world.

The immediate needs are often for security, food, shelter and healthcare. Local services are unable to respond to the rapid concentration of injured and often traumatised people. A large number of organisations—as listed in Chapter 7—are devoted to providing humanitarian assistance to those affected by these disasters. Many of these organisations need to deploy people at short notice and medical personnel are often amongst those who are in high demand.

Humanitarian assistance is by definition different from development work (covered in more detail in Chapter 13), which tries to address the underlying socio-political and economic factors that prevent the long-term development of a community or nation.

As many health workers toy with the idea of putting their skills to good use during emergencies, we have dedicated this short chapter to specifically exploring humanitarian relief. It aims to help you to understand whether this demanding type of work is for you.

A brief introduction

The Centre for Research on the Epidemiology of Disasters defines a *disaster* as 'a situation or event that overwhelms local capacity, necessitating a request to a national or international level for external assistance'. An *emergency* is when the crude mortality rate (CMR) is greater than 1 death per 10,000 people per day. If the CMR doubles, this is classified as an *acute emergency* (http://www.cred.be).

The number of natural disasters is on the rise, in contrast to disasters due to human conflict, which have decreased. Nevertheless, in regions or countries where human conflict continues, it is often protracted and takes an enormous toll on the population.

Key facts and figures on humanitarian disasters

Natural disasters:

- Natural disasters have almost trebled since the 1980s: from 140 in 1980 to 448 in 2007.
- Vast numbers of people are affected by disasters—2.54 million between 1997 and 2007.
- By 2015, over 375 million people per year are likely to be affected by climate-related disasters. This is 54% more than those affected in an average year during the last decade.

(Man-made) Conflict:

- There were over 14 million refugees in 2007.
- There are 26 million people displaced within their own countries by armed conflict.
- Conflicts fell by 40% between 1992 and 2004, but many remain, some even after a formal 'peace' deal has been agreed. The great majority of them are in poor countries.
- Worldwide, conflicts between armed groups declined by a third—from 36 to 24—between 2002 and 2006.

Source: *http://www.oxfam.org.uk/resources/issues/conflict/introduction.html*, last updated May 2009, reproduced with the permission of Oxfam GB, Oxfam House, John Smith Drive, Cowley, Oxford, OX4 2JY, UK. Oxfam does not necessarily endorse any text or activities that accompany the material.

Much of the focus of humanitarian work is in LMIC, as these countries are frequently affected by war and conflict and also disproportionately affected by natural disasters, as their investment in disaster preparedness is often minimal.

When a natural or man-made disaster strikes, the rest of the world usually responds with *humanitarian assistance*: the provision of material, logistics and human support 'to save lives, alleviate suffering and maintain human dignity'.

Some humanitarian organisations stop at this, while other organisations are involved in longer-term processes as well. These organisations stay on to try to ensure the sustainability of their interventions by supporting the rehabilitation and development

"Many people assume that they will be working in direct clinical care, but this is seldom the case except in acute emergency situations. The needs are more in building the capacity of the local staff through training and management in partnership with the Ministry of Health and local communities."

Nurse and midwife, Merlin

of local health systems. These organisations recruit health professionals on a longer-term basis to build capacity and sustain what has been achieved.

On some occasions, in 'chronic emergencies' like Eastern Congo or in certain areas like the Occupied Palestinian Territories, this is not possible. Here humanitarian agencies are unable to do anything except relief work because the pervasiveness of the conflict hinders or even prevents development agencies having any effective engagement or implementing development initiatives.

Organisations respond in different ways depending on the disaster and its location. For example, if an organisation is already working in the country where the disaster occurs, it is able to respond using local capacity. Additional emergency teams, extra staff and logistics will be sent up to boost the local response. The ability to respond depends on the staff available locally and internationally, as well as access to the disaster.

When several aid organisations, national and international, all rush to a disaster zone at the same time there can be huge problems of coordination and cooperation. In the past, rivalry between the organisations may have, on occasion, taken precedence over saving lives and alleviating suffering. In response to these problems, policies and processes have been implemented, such as the UN cluster system *(http://www.oneresponse.info/Pages/default.aspx)* and the Sphere project (see Box 8.1). However, emergency situations remain complex and challenging environments to work in.

Box 8.1: Best practice standards

These standards refer to the way humanitarian organisations should engage with one another and how they should treat their staff. It is important for you because this will indicate the professionalism of an organisation in the field, and what type of support you could expect from them to ensure your safety and training.

Humanitarian Accountability Partnership International (HAP International) was established in 2003 and is the humanitarian sector's first international self-regulatory body, working towards the promotion of 'humanitarian accountability'. *http://www.hapinternational.org*

The Code of Conduct for Red Cross and Red Crescent Movement and NGOs in Disaster Relief was developed and agreed upon by eight of the world's largest disaster response agencies in 1994. It is a voluntary code that sets the standards for organisations involved in humanitarian work. In 2007, there were more than 400 organisations signed up to it (IFRC 2007). *http://www.ifrc.org/en/publications-and-reports/code-of-conduct/*

The Sphere Project was launched in 1997 by a group of humanitarian NGOs and the Red Cross and Red Crescent movement. Its aim is to define and uphold the standards by which the global community responds to the plight of people affected by disasters, principally through a set of guidelines, known as the *Sphere Handbook*. *http://www.sphereproject.org*

The People in Aid Code of Good Practice is a management tool that helps humanitarian aid and development agencies enhance the quality of their human resources management. It helps to improve standards, accountability and transparency amid the challenges of disaster, conflict and poverty. *http://www.peopleinaid.org/code*

During armed conflicts, medical personnel, along with civilians and other groups of people who do not take part in the fighting, are protected by International Humanitarian Law (IHL). This gives them a legal guarantee that they must be protected and treated humanely in all circumstances. A major part of IHL is contained in the four Geneva Conventions of 1949. Nearly every state in the world has agreed to be bound by them. The law sets out a number of clearly recognisable symbols (the red cross and red crescent) which can be used to identify protected people, places and objects protected by IHL. Implementing the law is difficult during times of extreme violence and sadly there are cases where it is not respected.

Find out more

- IHL—the ICRC has a fact sheet *What Is International Humanitarian Law?* as well as much additional information on the subject. *http://www.icrc.org/ eng/assets/files/other/what_is_ihl.pdf*
- Humanitarian financing—where does the money come from and where does it go? Find out more from *http://www.globalhumanitarianassistance.org*, a website specifically dedicated to this.

Getting into the sector

"If someone is serious about this, they should recognise that there is a need for self-funded and self-supported training. You should train the same way you would train for your professional career in the UK."

Najeeb Rahman, Chairman, Doctors Worldwide

If you have little or no existing experience in international emergency work, breaking into the sector can be difficult. The number of people interested in this type of work outweighs demand. In order to get that first placement you need to stand out above the rest by showing enthusiasm and commitment, flexibility and adaptability. This will require an investment of time and money on your behalf. So, before doing this you need to consider carefully whether this type of work is for you.

"If you want fame and money, you are better off staying in the UK. Overseas work will not bring this."

Trauma surgeon, worldwide

Who do humanitarian organisations recruit?

In the initial stages of a crisis, most organisations will only recruit from a pool of experienced health professionals. Teamwork and self-sufficiency are vital and cannot easily be assessed in a recruitment process. You can't have loose cannons on a team in an emergency, as this could disrupt everyone's work. But as crises improve or stabilise, organisations may recruit less-experienced candidates.

The type of health professionals needed will depend on the nature of the next humanitarian crisis. Is it a famine, an epidemic or a war? And what stage is it at? A quick glance at the humanitarian organisations listed in Chapter 7 shows that within the health sector those in greatest demand are doctors and nurses (especially those who specialise in surgery, anaesthesia, reproductive health and psychiatry) along with midwives, epidemiologists, public health practitioners, nutritionists, water and sanitation engineers, and logisticians.

Most organisations require people to have a minimum of 2 years' post-qualification experience. So, if you are at the early stages of your career, not yet specialised and know you want to do emergency work, you could tailor your training towards one of these areas.

> "I dropped out of university at 20. I didn't know what to do, so I went travelling for 4 years. In 1999, I first heard of MSF and realised that I wanted to work with them.
>
> I didn't have the skills, so I came back to the UK to get my nursing training. I attended evening classes to learn French. Once I became a nurse, I enrolled for a Diploma in Tropical Nursing at LSHTM.
>
> I've been working with MSF since 2006, undertaking missions of 6–10 months in the Democratic Republic of Congo, Central African Republic and Sudan. I try to stay 2–3 months in the UK in between missions. I need it."
>
> *Nurse, MSF*

Personal characteristics and disposition are just as important as qualifications. The work and lifestyle are hard and the conditions can be tough. Self-reliance, resilience and good team skills are arguably the most important characteristics that you can offer. It is also extremely beneficial to have additional language skills.

Improve your chances of recruitment

Remember to think about the people you hope to work with, their situations and the professional and practical skills you will need to help them. The following list highlights some of the things you can do to make yourself stand out, helping you to make the transition from inexperienced to experienced emergency worker.

- Undertake one of the **introductory courses** on working in an emergency context (see Appendix 3).
- For doctors and nurses, consider a **diploma in tropical medicine/nursing**. An MSc in public health tends to be more applicable once you have gained some practical field experience. For nonclinicians, develop skills in bookkeeping, HR, accounting, supply and procurement, electrics, vehicle maintenance and administration.
- Gain experience of **working in resource-poor countries**, in a development rather than an emergency context, as this provides experience in a less tense environment. Whilst studying, electives can be an effective way to gain an initial insight into working in resource-poor settings.
- Focus on gaining **practical skills** rather than just academic qualifications. Core skills such as teaching, supervision, management and leadership are very useful. You could also undertake specialist assignments in project management or logistics.
- Become proficient in another **language**, e.g. French or Spanish.

The application process

Once you are confident that you have the appropriate professional skills and competence, along with some additional qualifications and experience under your belt that will help you to stand out, it is time to start the application process.

Identify and target organisations you want to work for. Attending events or careers fairs such as the NGO Forum (http://www.ngoforum.org.uk) is a good way to meet people who have been in the field and the pros and cons of different organisations. Chapter 7 also gives you an idea of some of the main organisations that work in emergency contexts and the criteria you might want to use before accepting a placement. This will help you to understand which organisations you are best suited to so you can target your applications. Some specific criteria you may want to use when applying to humanitarian organisations are:

- Their mission statement—does it resonate with you?
- Typical length of placement—does this fit with your availability?
- Geographical area and level of risk
- Pre-departure preparation, on-the-ground support and post-mission support offered
- Learning and development opportunities
- Possibilities for career development
- Conditions of respite breaks for longer assignments
- Adherence to standards for humanitarian assistance (see Box 8.1)
- Balance between humanitarian crisis and post-crisis development work.

Many organisations will have a rigorous recruitment process. Some organisations recruit for specific positions, while others will recruit people onto a database who are then called upon as and when needed, often at short notice.

If you are not recruited by an organisation, ask for feedback. Target your training and personal development, to ensure that you are more marketable in the future.

Preparation

Once you are accepted by an organisation and listed onto their database, be ready. It may be several months before you get called up, but when it does happen, you will probably only have 1 or 2 weeks' notice. When you have done a few assignments, you could be called up with only 24 hours' notice. Start preparing for your assignment in advance of being matched to a position.

If you are in a full-time job and wish to take time off to undertake humanitarian work, you should let your line manager know your intentions and negotiate time off work. In the NHS it is possible to take time out, but you will have to plan for this either as a sabbatical, unpaid leave or—for doctors in specialist training—taking time out of your training programme (OOP—see Chapter 4).

Find out more

For information on the options for taking time out of work to do humanitarian or development work refer to:
- *The DH Framework for NHS Involvement in International Development and International Humanitarian and Health Work: Tool Kit to Support Good Practice*
- The BMA's *Broadening Your Horizons* pamphlet: *Guidance for Doctors Taking Time Out to Work and Train in Developing Countries*
- The RCN/RCM leaflet *Working with Humanitarian Organisations: A Guide for Nurses, Midwives and Health Care Professionals*
- Consult with your Royal College as well, as they can provide useful information in this area.

The following chapter looks in detail at pre-departure preparation for any type of assignment. In addition, the following points are particularly relevant to humanitarian work:

- **Personal logistics:** Identify people to give as contacts in case of emergencies and officially name someone to act on your behalf for official business. Organise internet banking in advance and think about how you will make any loan, mortgage and rent payments.

- **Personal wellbeing:** Consider how you will manage this whilst you are overseas. Field work and living conditions can be extremely stressful, and it is useful to know how to unwind and relax so as to manage your stress levels and stay healthy. Build up a stock of books to take with you or invest in a Kindle. Buy in any essential items that you will need while away.
- **Health:** Ensure that all your vaccinations are up to date as shortened courses can be less effective for some vaccines than the usual longer courses. Keep your vaccination records safe, particularly your yellow fever certificate as this is required for entry into some countries. See your GP for a general health check as well, as you want to ensure that you are fit for the mission, and find out your blood group in case of emergency blood transfusions. Organise a dental check-up and any necessary treatment—this can potentially be very expensive and unpleasant whilst working overseas in remote areas.
- **Professional:** Make paper copies and scans of relevant diplomas (useful for visa applications and in the field). Make sure your professional body is aware of any change of address so that you don't miss any important communications from them.

What organisations may not tell you during briefings

Some unexpected problems may arise for which you were not prepared during briefing and training. Listed below are some of the surprising things for which people were not adequately prepared:

- Conflict between head office and the local offices of your organisation which might force your team to move from one area to another at short notice. This can impact on the sustainability of the organisation's work and your own role.
- Lack of coordination or even competition between international organisations. This can hinder your ability to deliver effective healthcare to the communities you are working with.
- Local organisations not being invited or refusing to attend meetings. This can make it difficult to work for or with them or to develop effective relationships.
- Problems liaising with the local health authorities and other political institutions, in particular in places where the government does not recognise your organisation.

Further opportunities

Working for an humanitarian organisation need not be a one-off *ad hoc* activity. If your first experience is a positive one, you will have to evaluate whether this is something you want to continue doing in future. Having experience in the field will make it easier for you to be recruited for placements.

If the latter is the case, you can contact your HR department again to look for another mission. It is also helpful to take some time out between missions, to ensure you are well rested and in good health before you take on a new challenge. It is not unusual to return home from a mission and find yourself overwhelmed with memories, thoughts and ideas, and you need time to process these. Taking a break also enables you to maintain links with family, friends and your profession.

"I would recommend developing a relationship with one organisation. Once you have done an overseas mission which has gone well and they know you, they are likely to call upon you for further assignments. Don't mess them around. Inform them when you are available and when you are not, and don't play them off against another organisation."

Careering humanitarian worker

If on the other hand you choose to resettle back at home, there is the opportunity to stay connected with organisations, both through the above mechanisms and by working in the humanitarian sector in the UK. See Chapter 15 for further details.

Conclusion

This chapter will have given you a snapshot of what humanitarian work is and how you can get into the sector. Chapter 11 looks in further detail at some of the specifics of working in humanitarian contexts, and covers issues such as security, health and safety, personal and professional challenges.

REFERENCE

IFRC (2007). *Code of Conduct*. http://www.ifrc.org/en/publications-and-reports/code-of-conduct.

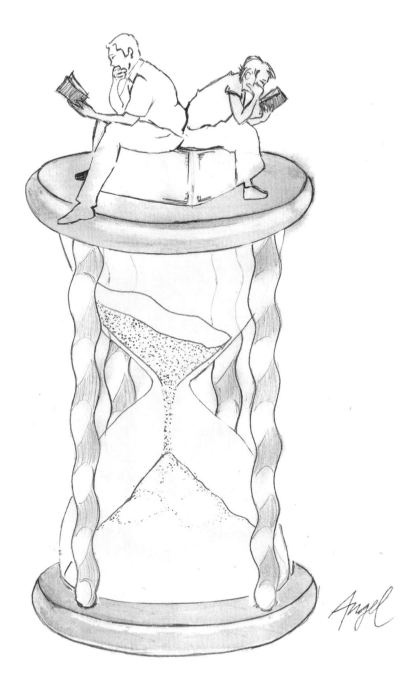

CHAPTER 9

Before you go

If you have arranged a placement overseas—congratulations! Now comes the rather more tedious time of preparing to go away. This can be a stressful period and tying up everything to go overseas often takes longer than expected. You may have anything from a few weeks to many months before your departure. In general, more preparation leads to a smoother placement. However, if you have only limited time available, this chapter will ensure you tick off the essentials.

The chapter is divided into three sections: **leaving your life behind** (dealing with UK professional issues), **preparing to work overseas** (professional issues in your host country) and **preparing to live overseas** (covering the more practical aspects of living in a different country). Of course, if you are only going on a short placement, then the longer-term aspects won't be as relevant, and you should concentrate on the second section. A checklist is provided at the end to make sure you have covered all points before departure.

Leaving your life behind

Registration here

There is no need to be registered with any of the UK regulatory bodies whilst you are practising overseas. You can apply for voluntary erasure whilst away, which will save you the annual retention fee. If you choose to remain registered, however, you will need to meet the normal registration requirements such as CPD evidence and meeting standards of practice.

At the end of your placement, you will need to restore your registration. This usually entails an application form, information about the work experience gained during your time away and letters of reference from your employers. If you have been registered with other professional councils overseas, you may require a 'Certificate of Good Standing' from them, which is a statement that you have not been subject to any fitness to practise investigations. Any 'return to practice' requirements only need to be met if you weren't practising whilst overseas for a substantial period.

Revalidation

The purpose of revalidation is to ensure that registered clinicians remain up to date and continue to be fit to practise. Revalidation is being considered by all the regulatory bodies and is likely to be a prerequisite for continued registration.

Revalidation will be introduced first by the GMC in 2012. Consultants and GPs will probably undergo revalidation every 5 years; therefore it will be most relevant to longer-term placements. Evidence of CPD and annual appraisals are likely to be counted towards revalidation, and thus building up a portfolio whilst overseas is essential (see Chapter 12).

Obtaining time out

Chapter 4 reviewed the possible ways to take time out of your NHS career. Here we describe how to formalise this time away.

NHS EMPLOYEES

If you're asking for a leave of absence, career break or sabbatical, talk to your line manager, head of department and HR department as early as possible. They will need to arrange for a replacement or locum cover, and will need plenty of notice.

A good way to get their endorsement is by sharing with them existing policy on support for international health work. The following documents contain information about the reciprocal benefits of getting involved in international health work for the UK and for people and health systems overseas, as well as endorsements from the DH in England, the NHS and NHS Employers:

- *Global Health Partnerships: The UK Contribution to Health in LMIC. http://www. dh.gov.uk*
- *Health is Global: Proposals for a UK Government-wide Strategy. http://www. dh.gov.uk*
- *The Framework for NHS Involvement in International Development. http:// www.ihlc.org*

Make sure that the necessary arrangements are in place for your re-entry into the UK workforce. See Chapters 12 & 14.

DOCTORS IN TRAINING

If you're in postgraduate medical training and are taking time out of your specialist training programme (OOP), then you need to decide whether you're applying for OOPE—out of programme experience—or OOPT—out of programme training. The latter will count towards your overall training time, but will need formal supervision and involves more work to arrange it. Talk to your educational supervisor and training programme director as soon as possible about your plans—they can help you with this decision.

You will need to fill out an OOP application form from your deanery, which needs to be signed by your educational supervisor and deanery representatives. The deanery will probably liaise directly with your medical college, but you should make sure the college is informed of your plans, one way or another.

For OOPE, once approval comes through, this is all you need to do for now. For OOPT, you will now need to get approval of your overseas work as training time. For this, you will need to get GMC approval. This can be quite arduous, so start early and be persistent.

The actual application is made through your deanery, but you will need to write a statement in support of your placement. The BMA publication *Broadening your Horizons* has template application letters. Try to include details on:

- Activities to be undertaken
- Supervisory arrangements
- Competencies and skills that you hope to gain
- Personal benefits

Once you have GMC approval, you will need to finalise your placement dates with your deanery.

Find out more

- *Broadening Your Horizons: A Guide to Taking Time Out to Work and Train in Developing Countries*. BMA International Department, March 2009. *http:// www.bma.org.uk/international/working_abroad/broadeningyourhorizons.jsp*
- *The Gold Guide: A Reference Guide for Postgraduate Specialty Training in the UK*. Medical Speciality Training (England), 2010. *http://www.mmc.nhs.uk/ specialty_training_2010/gold_guide.aspx*

Identify mentors and arrange appraisals

In Chapter 12, we outline the benefits of having both a UK and local mentor if possible. It is certainly easier to arrange your UK mentor now and agree a supervision schedule and personal development plan. Whilst it may be difficult to identify local mentors at this stage, it can make your first few weeks smoother if you can make arrangements before your departure.

Most NHS contracts stipulate that employees have an annual appraisal every 12 months (except those in training). If possible, try to undertake this shortly before you go away, as this provides a useful reference point for your employers when you return. If your appraisal falls during your time away, see if you can postpone it or ask your employers if your local or UK mentor could undertake it. An online appraisal toolkit such as at http://www.appraisals.nhs.uk could facilitate the process.

> **To think about**
>
> ....
>
> The DH (in England) maintains a database of volunteering organisations that it recognises for appraisal purposes. Individuals with registered organisations can undertake their annual appraisal whilst in placement. This is an excellent way of ensuring that their experience abroad is valued and integrated within the NHS. Check if your organisation is registered before you leave, and if not encourage them to sign up.

Personal finances

There are four main aspects to your personal finances that will be affected by time away: your NHS pension contributions (if applicable), National Insurance contributions, student loan repayments and income tax. You should also think about how you will access money abroad.

NHS PENSION CONTRIBUTIONS

If you want to make contributions whilst you are away, then you will need what is referred to as a Section 7(2) Direction. If your overseas employment is approved, then you will be able to continue making contributions into the NHS pension scheme. Section 7(2) Directions are granted automatically for DFID advisory posts, UN or WHO posts, and for certain British aid organisations such as Oxfam and Save the Children. Otherwise, you will need to apply for your own Direction, which is assessed on a case-by-case basis by the NHS Pensions Agency. Essentially, your work overseas will need to be for a limited time (i.e. you can't continue to pay in if your whole career is overseas), for charitable purposes, and your last NHS employer will need to sponsor your application.

VSO and the British Red Cross already hold their own Section 7(2) Directions. Therefore any NHS pension scheme member going to work abroad with these organisations can apply to remain within the scheme.

If you get your own Direction, then you will have to pay both your own and your employer contributions based on your last NHS salary. The NHS Pensions Agency will invoice you, and you will need to pay them directly by cheque or standing order.

> **Find out more**
>
> ....
>
> • Appendix 2 of the NHS Pension Scheme (DH_5044914). *http://www.dh.gov.uk*
> • Talk to your NHS pensions officer

NATIONAL INSURANCE CONTRIBUTIONS

To decide whether to make voluntary contributions, get a Pensions Forecast from Directgov (http://www.direct.gov.uk/pensions). This will tell you whether making voluntary contributions will boost your basic State Pension and what you will have to pay to make up your missing contributions. You can pay by direct debit whilst you're away or up to six tax years following the tax year in which you missed contributions.

Find out more

....

- *HMRC leaflet NI38: Social Security Abroad. http://www.hmrc.gov.uk*
- National Insurance: *http://www.direct.gov.uk/nationalinsurance*

STUDENT LOAN REPAYMENTS

A student loan, if you have one, is usually administered through the UK tax system by the Student Loans Company (SLC).

If you are going abroad for more than 3 months, contact SLC as soon as possible to inform them of your circumstances. If you are volunteering, then you won't have to make any repayments as you won't have any income. If you are earning, then you can make student loan repayments directly to SLC whilst you are overseas—either by monthly direct debit or in a lump sum payment when you return. The type of loan you have will determine your repayment amount, but the repayment thresholds are different in other countries in order to take account of differences in living costs. The repayment thresholds for different countries can be found at http://www. studentloanrepayment.co.uk.

INCOME TAX

You can apply for a tax rebate as soon as you receive your last payslip before your time away, or on your return. The amount you will get back depends on a number of factors, including:

- How long you spend abroad
- Whether you will be abroad for a complete financial year
- Who your employer is—UK-based (e.g. Merlin) or overseas
- Taxation practice in your destination country

The easiest way to find out whether you're entitled to anything is to contact your local tax office (there's a locator on the HMRC website http://www.hmrc.gov.uk) and outline your situation. You will need to send in copies of your P60/P45 forms for the tax year for which you're claiming (the tax year runs 6 April to 5 April) and also any relevant documents about your employment that year (both UK and overseas). From 2012, you will have up to 4 years to claim retrospectively.

Remember that you might also be eligible for a rebate on your council tax—contact your council directly.

ACCESSING MONEY ABROAD

It is unwise to carry large amounts of cash as it could get stolen. In some countries (although the number is reducing) it is difficult to use international cards at cash machines, although usually money can be withdrawn at the bank. You should tell your UK bank and credit card company that you will be withdrawing money overseas and from which countries, otherwise they may freeze your account on suspicion of fraud (it has happened to the authors numerous times!).

You might want to consider opening an account abroad either for personal use or to channel funds to support the project that you are involved with. You can do this from the UK, but it is preferable to do it in person when you get there. Get recommendations from colleagues and friends about banks, and check these banks on the internet to find out about fee charges for money transfers and other facilities. To open the bank account in person you will usually need to have passport photos, proof of local address and one or two local references. You might also need to bring with you a local utility bill.

Transferring money overseas from the UK can be very expensive. Some banks charge a flat fee of up to £50 per transfer. There are, thankfully, some cheaper ways of doing it. Consider setting up a PayPal account before you leave. People in the UK can pay into this account for a fraction of the cost of bank transfers. You can then make a withdrawal from your PayPal account into your bank account for a small fee (http://www.paypal.co.uk).

Also consider a money transfer company such as Western Union. Shop around, though, as the fees and exchange rates vary considerably. Exchange rates are going to become very important when you're abroad. Many currencies in LMIC countries experience continuous fluctuations throughout the year. Keep an eye on the current exchange rate and try to receive money from the UK when the pound is strong. You can compare money transfer companies and sign up to an exchange rate alert at http://www.comparemoneytransfer.com.

Preparing to work overseas

Registration there

Registration requirements vary from country to country. If you're going with an organisation, they will usually sort this out for you.

If you're going on your own, you will need to contact the relevant professional association in your host country to check the requirements and submit any documentation necessary. Your professional association or regulatory body might be able to help you identify the correct counterpart in your host country. Failing that, *The Medic's Guide to Work and Electives Around the World* (Wilson 2009) lists many professional councils in individual countries for doctors, nurses, dentists and physiotherapists.

You will usually need official copies of your qualifications and registration. Sometimes this has to be notarised, which can be very expensive, so make sure you have all the right documents to minimise the number of visits. Your regulatory body should also be able to provide you with a Certificate of Good Standing (see above). If you intend to prescribe during your placement, check with the local medical council directly that you will have the legal right to do so in that country.

Indemnity insurance

If you're going with an organisation, check that they have an indemnity policy to cover your work overseas with them. If they don't and you need to go through your own provider, your organisation might cover a percentage or all the costs and should be able to provide you with an appropriate risk assessment.

If you have arranged your own placement, phone your current indemnity provider. Many trips will be covered on a discretionary basis, but you must have this in writing before you leave. See Box 9.1 for the policies of the three main medical defence organisations. If they can't insure you, they can usually recommend an insurance broker. Having official documents about your placement and a signed letter from overseas requesting your services might come in handy for this discussion.

Travel and medical insurance

If you're going with an organisation, travel and medical insurance will usually be provided by them. However, make sure you have adequate cover for any travelling you might do in your free time.

If you're making your own arrangements, standard insurance policies will only cover certain countries and for a set duration. If you are on a medium- or long-term placement or going to a high-risk area, you will need specific, higher-cover insurance. For high-risk areas, check that your destination is covered and that the policy includes evacuations, hijack/kidnap and conflict situations. THET has a useful summary of aspects to consider (http://www.thet.org/practical-information/).

Passport

Many countries will not accept passports with less than 6 months' remaining validity on them. The FCO website (http://www.fco.gov.uk) lists the requirement for individual countries. Make sure you also have several blank pages in case you need a visa both for your destination country and for travelling whilst you're out there. If you still have

> **Box 9.1: Medical defence organisations' policies on working overseas**
>
> ....
>
> **Medical Protection Society (MPS)** (*http://www.medicalprotection.org/uk*)
>
> If you plan to work overseas you must contact the MPS well in advance of your trip, to ensure that you have appropriate indemnity arrangements. This is particularly important because some countries have made it a requirement that all healthcare practitioners have insurance-based indemnity, as discretionary indemnity is not recognised in these areas. The MPS is the world's largest mutual medical protection organisation working internationally, operating in more than 40 countries. If you are planning to work overseas, you may well be able to continue your membership with them.
>
> **Medical Defence Union (MDU)** (*http://www.the-mdu.com/*)
>
> Members are advised to contact the MDU to discuss their plans before departure as their subscriptions and any benefits available will be dependent on the location and the nature of the work. If you are in a training grade in the UK and a paying member of the MDU you are entitled to be covered under the professional indemnity insurance policy for work of up to 1 year in a recognised supervised training post overseas (except in the United States, Canada, Bermuda, Israel, Hong Kong, Australia and Zimbabwe). This does not cover clinical work undertaken in a private or unsupervised capacity overseas. The MDU can provide discretionary indemnity for doctors who are not in training grades and who are looking to work overseas for no more than 3 months, for example teaching or working for a charity. Whatever you intend to do, you will need to contact the MDU before you go and on your return.
>
> **Medical and Dental Defence Union of Scotland (MDDUS)** (*http://www.mddus.com/*)
>
> Members are advised to contact the membership department before leaving the UK. Paid employment overseas is not covered, but voluntary work with UK-registered charities is covered.

time remaining on your current passport and decide to renew, then the validity of your new passport can be extended to include the unexpired time from your old one.

If you're in a hurry, the Identity and Passport Service offers a fast-track 1-week and even a 1-day renewal service, but you'll need to go to a regional passport office and it will cost you. See http://www.ips.gov.uk for more information.

It's a good idea to have a copy of your passport in case of loss. Even better than a paper copy is scanning and emailing it to yourself and a relative.

Visas

The Foreign Office website lists the visa requirements for British nationals by country (http://www.fco.gov.uk). Obtaining visas takes time and money–so start early. If your visit is last minute, you can often get fast-track visas for a fee. Indeed, some travel companies offer this service, saving you the hassle of queuing up at the embassy. For medium- and long-term placements, you will require a work visa. In most cases you apply for this once in the country and enter on a tourist or business visa. Check the requirements with the country embassy or consulate here as you will often need supporting documentation, for example a UK criminal record bureau check, copies of your degree certificates and a letter from your employer.

> ### Elective Advice
>
> ....
>
> The RCN International Department offers useful advice which is applicable to all electives:
>
> "If you put in your visa application that you want to 'work' or do 'work experience' in the host country, it may be assumed that you are looking for paid work and this can delay your visa. It is better to state that you would like to spend time in a healthcare setting in the host country as part of your course of higher education in the UK."

Register with your embassy

All British embassies offer a registration service called LOCATE for all British nationals visiting or living in a foreign country. This means that embassy and emergency staff can give you better assistance in a crisis such as a tsunami or terrorist attack. Once you register, you can update your details for any future trips or once you have a local phone number. It's easiest to register online at http://www.fco.gov.uk/locateportal.

In case you cannot register online, go to the British Embassy or High Commission upon arrival. In the case where there is no UK representation in the country you will be staying in, you should find out whether registration at another EU country office is possible. All EU countries have reciprocal arrangements with each other.

Train up

If you're going with an organisation, they are likely to offer you training before your departure in topics such as security, personal health, project management, needs assessment and managing a team.

If you're going on your own, you may want to get some of this training yourself. Both RedR (http://www.redr.org.uk) and Interhealth (http://www.interhealth.org.uk) offer London-based training courses with places for individuals.

Whether you're going on your own or not, review your skill set in light of your placement and likely case-mix. Many of our case studies emphasised the importance of doing a tropical medicine/nursing course and gaining appropriate emergency life support skills: see Appendix 3.

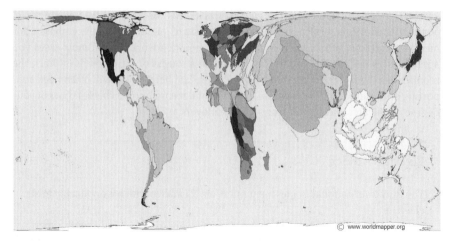

Figure 9.1 Map of global road deaths, 2001. (Territory size shows the proportion of all road traffic accident deaths worldwide that occurred in that territory.) © Copyright SASI Group (University of Sheffield).

Driving

Remember that road traffic accidents are one of the biggest killers of British nationals abroad (see Figure 9.1).

If you will be driving abroad, check whether you will need an International Driving Permit in your host country. This allows the holder to drive a private motor vehicle with a valid UK driving licence. Such permits are valid for 12 months from the date of issue and can be obtained by post or from the Post Office. There are different requirements according to country—see http://www.theaa.com/motoring_advice/overseas.

Try to find out the driving laws of your host country in advance, including local speed limits and blood alcohol limits, either through their embassy or your contacts.

If you will be driving for work, then you should check with your indemnity and travel insurance providers that you will be fully covered for these periods, including medical expenses resulting from any accidents.

Finally, consider an off-road driving course if you will be driving over rough terrain or stationed in a rural/remote area. These courses cover techniques to drive safely through mud, sand, water and on steep inclines and will reduce the likelihood of both accidents and damage to your vehicle. The website http://www.ukoffroad.com lists course providers around the UK.

Health

Try not to leave this until the last minute. Your GP might be able to provide some of the medication below, but if not contact your nearest travel clinic. If you work for the NHS, find out what support you can get from your NHS occupational health department. Find out about common diseases in the country and region you are going to and local healthcare facilities near the place you will be working. This will help you prepare your first-aid kit.

> ### Find a travel clinic close to you
> ....
> - The British Travel Health Association: *http://www.bhta.org/travel_clinic_directory.asp*
> - TravelHealth.co.uk: *http://www.travelhealth.co.uk/travelclinics*

HIV POST-EXPOSURE PROPHYLAXIS (PEP)

If you are undertaking clinical practice and could get a needlestick injury, then you should take an HIV PEP pack. These tend to contain about a week's worth of prophylaxis and can usually be bought from your UK occupational health department (or will be provided by your organisation). If you do get a needlestick injury, you are likely to have to make the risk assessment yourself about whether it is worth starting the prophylaxis course, bearing in mind the specifics of the injury and the local HIV prevalence (so find this out in advance). You will then need to liaise with a medical service somewhere regarding whether to continue the course and make arrangements for follow-up testing (Wilson 2009).

VACCINES

Courses of most travel vaccines can be administered over a 4-week period. The final doses should ideally be completed a little ahead of the departure date to allow full immunity to develop. If you need any primary courses of vaccines rather than boosters, then more time will be required. If the full course cannot be completed before your departure date, then it is usually worth having the maximum number of doses possible, and completing the course on your return (National Travel Health Network and Centre 2010).

Rabies vaccine is recommended if you are likely to be in contact with domestic animals, particularly dogs, or other rabies vectors such as bats or foxes in an endemic country.

Yellow fever is now the only disease for which an international vaccination certificate may be required for entry into a country. This is valid for 10 years beginning 10 days after the vaccination date. Keep your certificate safe in your hand luggage. Keep a photocopy of the certificate, as if you lose it your practice can re-issue it.

The WHO International Travel and Health Interactive map gives individual country information on yellow fever requirements, malaria risk and recommended prophylaxis, and rabies risk (http://apps.who.int/tools/geoserver/www/ith/index.html).

MALARIA PREVENTION

Malaria chemoprophylaxis is recommended in endemic areas to be used in conjunction with bite prevention (using repellents and insecticides, sleeping under an insecticide-treated net, using long trousers and shirts after dusk). Check which is the right antimalarial for your area. Remember that most courses need to be started slightly before travel. Mosquito nets and repellents can often be purchased locally at a fraction of the UK price, but if you are going to a remote area you may want to check with colleagues.

Build up your knowledge base

Now that you know your destination, do read up on it—including its health indicators and political context. This is as important as practical training in order to hit the ground running. The WHO country profiles (http://www.who.int/gho/countries), *CIA World Factbook* (http://www.cia.gov) and WHO regional office websites (listed in Chapter 6) are good places to start. You may also want to look at the Ministry of Health website if available for that country. The FCO (http://www.fco.gov.uk) has updates on the security situation in individual countries. You may also find it useful to know which organisations are working in the country or region and their projects (http://www.devdir.org).

If you're going with an organisation, go over its policies in depth. Try to find out as much as possible about your intended role and project, and arrangements on the ground, e.g. accommodation. If you're going on your own, try to talk to other health professionals who have worked or lived in the region to get a flavour of the working culture and common problems.

Prepare yourself for your first impressions

As you read more, the reality of the situation in your host country might seem overwhelming, but preparation can help you reduce the shock of the first few days. Doing some of the following things can be useful:
- Reading novels set in the country or non-fiction books about its history or current issues
- Watching relevant documentaries or films about life in the country to get a feel for the place
- Visiting blogs on the country, especially by people who live there, as they might discuss some of the issues you will face
- Reading local newspapers online
- Attending lectures on the country, where you can meet people with relevant experience and pick up useful tips

---

Prepare a risk assessment

This contextual information will help you develop your own risk assessment. It is essential that you know how to prepare for and mitigate potential risks, and make plans to deal with them if they happen.

Try to keep a checklist with details of the following: weather patterns and climate, the local gastronomy, availability of drinking water, public transport and personal safety, emergency measures such as repatriation procedures, local places of refuge such as churches and parish offices, and local police. This risk assessment can help when you talk to insurance brokers.

What to take for work

It is wise to start by finding out about your airline baggage allowance. Can you get any extra benefits as a result of your humanitarian work? Depending on the length of your placement, you might want to send some of your luggage in advance, in particular heavy items such as books and teaching aids. DHL Global Forwarding offers preferential shipping rates for health professionals involved in Health Links and international health work. Find out more at http://www.ihlc.org.uk.

Find out more

....

- THET and DHL fact sheet on shipping overseas *http://www.thet.org/practical-information*

When going to work in a resource-poor environment, it's natural to think about equipment and drugs that you could take with you to donate. However, short-term supplies can actually do more harm than good in the long-term. Do take anything you need to perform your job well (e.g. formularies, supply of disposable gloves), but read the section on equipment and drug donations in Chapter 11 before packing anything else.

If you are teaching, make sure you talk to your local contacts about teaching aids. Will you need them? What exactly should you take with you? Your contacts can also help you with local dress code and items that are difficult to obtain locally.

Preparing to live overseas

Communications

You are likely to need to communicate with local contacts before your departure and inform family members on how they can contact you. Remember that emails can be difficult to access locally, so don't rely on them alone. Follow-up with phone calls where possible.

Thankfully, the days of costly and poor quality long-distance phone calls are gone, and mobile technology is very popular in LMIC. There are now a variety of ways to stay in touch with your support network and work colleagues back home. Here are a few tips:

- Set up a **Skype** account (http://www.skype.com) and give your Skype name to your contacts. This is a software application that allows users to make voice calls over the internet. These are free to other Skype users or you can buy credit to make cheap calls.

- Email accounts accessed through secure sites (such as workplace accounts) can be difficult to get into at internet cafes. It's worth setting up a **generic email account**, such as Googlemail, Yahoo or Hotmail, and redirecting your emails there whilst you're away.
- Look up some **websites providing cheap telephone calls** over the internet, both to landlines and mobiles (for example, http://www.telediscount.co.uk and http://www.dialtosave.co.uk). Give the access numbers to your contacts here and take a cheap mobile out with you. When you arrive, buy a local SIM card and send your new number to your contacts. They can then phone you cheaply on your local mobile via the website's access numbers.

Personal relationships

It's worth having a think about relationships before you leave. Entering into a relationship with a local person during your placement can be complicated and may even jeopardise your work. Think about the power dynamics at play and if the person is vulnerable. How will you or your partner be perceived locally? What will happen at the end of your placement? Also remember that many cultures are not as liberal about sexual relationships as Europe and America. Having said that, many relationships do work out, but it's probably worth waiting until you're familiar with local cultural norms (Bolton and Welty 2006).

If you are gay, be aware that homosexuality is illegal in many countries. The FCO website lists attitudes towards homosexuality on its individual country pages (http://www.fco.gov.uk). Be mindful of relationships with local people, as they may be at more risk than you of violence or being shunned by their community.

Finally, the prevalence of sexually transmitted infections including HIV/AIDS is often higher than in the UK. Make sure you take some condoms from the UK, as those bought overseas can be of poor quality.

What to take to live

Although well-practised at critical decisions, the final packing session before a long trip abroad will test any health professional's decision-making skills. Limited space and a huge range of potential items to take will make the task feel like trying to square a circle. We polled our case studies for their top items to take with them overseas. We received quite a varied list as well as explanations, but they generally fell into three categories: body, soul and practicalities.

BODY

- Any medications you need for pre-existing conditions
- Preferred brand of sanitary towels/tampons or consider taking with you the Mooncup menstrual cup (http://www.mooncup.co.uk)
  - "But be prepared to explain what tampons are when you cross borders. There were some very suspicious male Brazilian guards and my limited tourist Spanish really wasn't up to the job"

- Contact lenses and solution
- Deodorant
- Lip balm
- Tweezers
  - "Very hard to describe in pidgin French"
- Appropriate clothing to suit the temperature and occasion
  - "In many countries appearance is more highly valued than in the UK. Just because you are in a poor country, don't switch your shirt for a scruffy t-shirt"

SOUL

- iPod and books/Kindle
  - "Especially if you are going to a remote area with little entertainment"
- Photos from home
- A decent radio
  - "If you are going for long periods of time and want the World Service to provide news from Blighty"
- Hard sweets which won't melt
- Creature comforts like Marmite or dark chocolate
- Balsamic vinegar
  - "If you get bored of goat stew and fancy doing something homely with a tomato"

PRACTICALITIES

- A voltage regulator
  - "Currency fluctuation can cause havoc to electrical equipment, especially laptop batteries. The regulator helps you keep a constant voltage level and will help maintain your appliances"
- An eco-friendly fold-away bag
  - "Plastic bags are now banned at markets in some countries like Rwanda and Bangladesh"
- A cotton white coat, especially for electives
  - "Clinicians in other countries may wear them far more than here and the heavier ones we can buy in the UK are stifling in the tropics. You can also get one made up cheaply as soon as you arrive"
- Swiss Army knife
- Travel plug
- A sarong
  - "One of the most multi-purpose items ever invented"
- Torch, ideally solar or wind-up
- A sleeping bag liner
  - "Makes almost any bed bearable"
- And finally, "common-sense"!

However, the absolute number-one item was a **portable laptop**. This combines entertainment, communications, photos and work. Moreover, with solar chargers and external hard drives, the practical drawbacks are no longer as relevant.

> ### Stuff your rucksack
>
> In the unlikely event that you have a few spare inches left over, think about *http://www.stuffyourrucksack.com*. This is a great initiative set up by the TV presenter Kate Humble in order to promote direct action for small projects, schools and charities overseas. The organisation will put their request on the website (inexpensive items such as pens, a world map, footballs), you check the list for your destination country, buy the items and deliver them to the project when you go out. Simple, and a great way to meet local people before you start work.

Conclusion

The pre-departure period will always be stressful, but we hope this chapter will ensure that the most essential aspects are covered. Think about it as part of your placement and this might help you enjoy it more. With these tedious chores completed, you will soon be stepping onto the plane to begin your exciting placement. The next section, In the Field, leads you through the settling-in process, how to get the most out of your placement, and the reality of working in international health.

REFERENCES

Bolton M, Welty E (2006). Surviving as an aid worker. *Working Abroad* 70 (September/October).

National Travel Health Network and Centre (2010). *Health Information for Overseas Travel (the 'Yellow Book')*. London: Department of Health.

Wilson M (2009). *The Medic's Guide to Work and Electives Around the World*, 3rd edition. London: Hodder Arnold.

The essential pre-departure checklist

HERE   COMPLETED

- Registration ☐
- Obtain approved time out ☐
- Pension contributions ☐
- National Insurance contributions ☐
- Student loan repayments ☐
- Set up a PayPal account ☐
- Identify UK mentor ☐
- Arrange appraisal ☐

THERE

- Registration ☐
- Passport and visa ☐
- Indemnity ☐
- Insurance ☐
- Register with LOCATE service ☐
- Make a risk assessment ☐
- International driving permit ☐
- Vaccines ☐
- Malaria prophylaxis ☐
- HIV post-exposure prophylaxis ☐
- Communications, e.g. Skype account ☐
- Identify local mentor. ☐

In the field

After all the preparation and packing, you're finally there. The smells are different, the sounds are different, and the work is very definitely different. Although exhilarating and absorbing, it also requires a great deal of adjustment on your part. If you are experiencing problems, the chances are other people have faced them as well—and got through it. In this section, we distil this learning into top pointers for getting to grips with your new environment.

Chapter 10 (Settling in) leads you through the process of adjustment, including the first few days and starting at work. This is a chapter to read before you go, but also to refer back to during the inevitable low points.

Chapter 11 (At work) describes the common constraints of resource-poor settings and differences in working practices, and how best to work within them.

In **Chapter 12 (Getting the most out of it)**, we look at how to maximise your professional development overseas, and use it to smooth your transition back into UK working life.

Lastly, **Chapter 13 (Making an impact)** concentrates on the enduring effect of your time abroad. Will the service function after you leave? Who will take over from you? Essentially, has your contribution been sustainable?

The final section **Coming home** focuses on winding up your placement and coming back to the reality of UK life and work. Although the immediate adventure may be over, we go through ways to make sense of your experiences and to stay involved in international work.

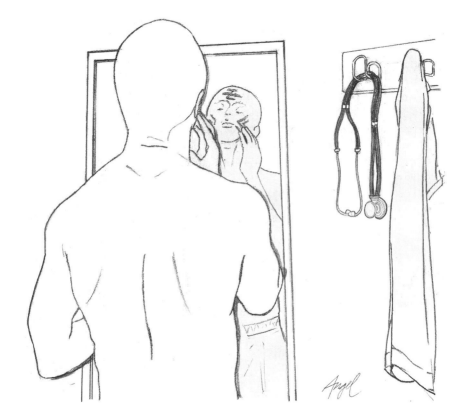

CHAPTER 10

Settling in

You have finally arrived at your destination. It may have been a frustrating trip, with everything from lost baggage to missed connections thrown your way. Finally reaching your host country will undoubtedly revive your spirits. It is extremely exciting to be outside of your normal routines in a completely different culture, and you may enter a honeymoon period with your new location.

But the initial excitement may wear off after a few days or weeks, and disillusionment or homesickness may take its place. Conditions and values can be very different to what is familiar, and the transition will take some adjustment.

This chapter takes you through some common problems that may arise during your settling-in period, and ways in which you can overcome these initial difficulties. These problems mainly affect those on mid- to long-term placements, but we have included some pointers for those on short placements as well.

Timeline for settling in

Adjusting to a new environment is a gradual process. Initial excitement soon gives way to the challenges of daily life in a different culture. You may start feeling irritated or resentful at things you could take for granted back in the UK. These feelings resolve with time for most people, but you are likely to have peaks and troughs of morale throughout your first 6 months. The timeline shown in Table 10.1 outlines typical phases for adjusting to a new culture.

As time passes, you will become more familiar with your new culture and find it easier to interpret the subtle cultural cues. You will feel more confident, develop new friends and manage social and professional interactions more comfortably.

Table 10.1 Phases of adjustment

Time period	General attitude and feelings	Emotional responses to events	Behavioural responses to events	Physical responses to events
At home	Anticipation	Excitement, enthusiasm, some fear of unknown, concern about leaving family, home and friends	Anticipation, loss of interest in current activities	Weariness, normal health
1 month	Exhilaration	Sense of mission and purpose tourist enthusiasm	Curiosity about nationals, avoidance of negative stereotypes	Intestinal disturbances, minor insomnia
2 months	Bewilderment, restlessness, impatience, disenchantment	Qualms, uncertainty, search for familiar activities, some withdrawal, increase in alcohol consumption	Neutral toward environment, scepticism, frustration, question values of others and self, much stress on family members	Colds, headaches
3 months	Discouragement, irritability	Discouragement, bewilderment, concerns about sanitation, homesickness	Avoid contact with local people, withdraw, fear of theft and injury, invoke stereotypes	Minor illnesses
4/5 months	Gradual recovery	Interest in new activities or cultural resignation	Constructive attitudes, accommodations	Normal health
6 months	Normal	Equilibrium	Equilibrium	Normal health

(Adapted from University of Michigan International Center, used with permission)

The first few days

These will usually be taken up with briefings and some more travelling if your final destination is a remote location.

Lack of sleep, jet lag and new surroundings may combine to leave you feeling extremely disorientated. You may experience a dip in morale and question your reasons for coming out. Remember that getting to your final base and unpacking will make you feel much more settled. Although culture shock tends to manifest later on, you may be susceptible if you have little experience of low-income settings.

The climate and altitude may affect you physically, so take it easy and give your body time to adjust. In hot climates keep yourself hydrated and out of the sun. Once acclimatised, water requirements increase rather than decrease, so maintain an adequate fluid intake.

> "As we only had 2 weeks, I wanted to fit as much in as possible and began 8 hours of operating each day. The theatre had little ventilation and I was operating in thick canvas gowns. I could feel the sweat pouring off me and I just couldn't rehydrate quickly enough in the evenings. After 2 days, I went down with heat stroke and had to take a few days out to recover, which was frustrating."
>
> *Consultant surgeon, Sierra Leone*

If feasible, consider arriving a week or so before the start of your official placement. This will allow you to absorb some of the culture and customs, and also try out some of your local phrases before having to use them in the workplace. The more cultural adjustment done now means the more you can concentrate on new working practices when you start your placement.

Short-term placements

If your placement is less than 1 month, you risk trying to fit in too much work, leaving little for adjustment. To maximise productivity, do timetable some free time at the start and mid-way through your placement for recuperation. The section below on starting at work is also relevant.

Jet lag

If you are to perform skilled tasks during your placement, then it is essential to plan in some time to recover from jetlag and lack of sleep. Adaptation to eastward travel generally takes longer than westwards. Rehydrate on the flight, avoid alcohol and eat lightly.

Melatonin supplements seem to be remarkably effective in preventing and reducing jet lag, especially if you are crossing five or more time zones. Occasional use appears safe (Herxheimer and Petrie 2009).

Common problems in the first few days

CHANGES TO YOUR JOB DESCRIPTION

You may arrive in the country to find that your job description is different to what you expected or even a completely different post. There are usually valid reasons for these changes. Organisations need to prioritise their resources, and this includes you. So unexpected circumstances may mean that you are re-allocated to a more vital project, even if this means some last-minute adjustment.

If, due to changes or miscommunication, the job differs substantially to your current competencies or the supervision level is far lower than what you feel comfortable with, then you must discuss this urgently with your organisation and line manager. It is better that you are comfortable and productive, rather than out-of-your-depth, potentially unsafe and unhappy.

ILLNESS

Common problems overseas are covered briefly in most guidebooks and extensively in the *Yellow Book* (Department of Health 2010), and of course complemented by your own knowledge.

Diarrhoea, heatstroke and sunburn are frequent early problems. Apart from minor problems, it is better and more professional to be diagnosed by someone else. Seek help early, especially if you are in doubt over your diagnosis. Local clinicians will have seen malaria a thousand times—you may have only seen it once.

The first month

This is the time to orient yourself to your immediate surroundings. You will need to know the local eateries, transport routes and the nearest hospital with emergency facilities. Also take the time to seek out some oases of Western culture, e.g. a coffee shop, sports club or cinema. Although you will probably want to immerse yourself now, it is likely that there will come a time when you will need a 'fix' of your home culture to get over a twinge of homesickness.

Security

Safety is an important aspect of settling in. You may have already had pre-departure briefings on security, but add to these by gathering local opinions regarding safety levels and crime hotspots. In most countries, walking in isolated places after dark is probably best avoided unless you know the area well. Be careful with your alcohol intake as excess could make you vulnerable.

> "I am very used to being independent, and walking everywhere. However, it was simply too dangerous to do so alone in my neighbourhood, even for someone who lives in south London. I had to get taxis everywhere,

⟳

which was frustrating and a big adjustment for me. Most men carried some form of weapon, which made me very uncomfortable coming from the UK. In fact, I was at a staff party once and was trying to open a bottle of vodka. Another guest offered to help me—by taking his gun out and trying to blow off the top of the bottle!"

Emergency doctor, Guyana

As with any trip abroad, there are a few golden rules (http://www.fco.gov.uk):

- Think about what you are doing at all times and trust your instincts—don't take risks that you wouldn't at home
- Don't openly display valuables such as mobile phones or digital cameras and consider using a padlock on suitcases and backpacks
- Find out about local laws—there may be serious penalties for breaking a law that might seem trivial at home

Cultural differences

Differences between the new culture and your home country may require early adaptation from you—especially if you are being welcomed by your hosts. Although assimilating this new culture can require a lot of energy, flexibility and patience from you, it is worth the investment as it can avoid much unintentional offence during your work.

"I was working in an area where Oshiwambo was the native language. In this culture how you greet people is very important. This was the first thing I was taught in my language lessons. The greeting involve a series of phrases going back and forth between two people asking about how the person is, how they slept and answering appropriately. Although this took time with a large group, it did enable me to gain respect amongst the local people, even if they laughed at some of my pronunciation!"

NHS manager, Namibia

Below are some specific pointers when working in a Muslim country/environment.

When working in a Muslim country

Clothing: both men and women should dress modestly. Women should wear long-sleeved tops and trousers or long skirts. Avoid low-cut tops and anything tight fitting or revealing. In more conservative countries, women should also wear a loosely fitting head scarf. Men should not wear shorts or rolled-up trousers. Long-sleeved shirts are best.

➲

General behaviour: when meeting people of the opposite sex, do not automatically offer a hand shake as this may cause offence. Take your cue from the people around you and see how they behave. It is fine for men to shake hands with other men, while women may do this with other women or offer two kisses to other women.

Avoid situations where you are alone with a person of the opposite sex, especially in your home and try to have a same-sex chaperone. Do not be overly friendly with someone of the opposite sex as this could be misinterpreted.

If alcohol is available, do not drink it in public places.

When examining patients of the opposite sex: always offer the patient a doctor/nurse of the same sex if they are available. If you are a woman, always have a chaperone present when examining a male patient. Be aware that they may not want to take their clothes off in front of you. A male doctor should try to avoid seeing a female patient alone. Always have another female health worker present and leave intimate examinations to a female doctor if possible. Often husbands will want to be present too.

Religion

Religion can pose particular difficulties, especially if you are not practising or non-religious. Many countries that require health workers are much less secular than the UK, and you are likely to be asked about your religion. It is worth thinking in advance how you intend to answer this question. If you are religious, joining a local place of worship can help you become part of the local community and be a source of great support and friends during your time abroad.

Languages

If you have taken the brave step of working in a different language, there are likely to be teething problems as you adjust to the local terminology and accent. Have patience—the day will come when it all clicks into place.

Even if you are working in an English-speaking country, there can be language difficulties. Thickly accented or pidgin English can be tough to get your head around, and your British accent may be incomprehensible to locals. Over time you will learn to modify your accent and use local phrases in order to maximise communication. See our top ten tips for communicating in English abroad, in the box below. Everyday gestures and body language may be different as well (e.g. a nod may not mean a nod).

In a country with many local languages, often only those who have attended secondary or higher education will speak the official language to a good level. Speaking to your healthcare colleagues usually isn't a problem, but it may be more difficult communicating with patients, local support staff and those you interact with daily, such as market sellers.

Efforts to learn common words and phrases in the local language will make your life much easier and are sure to be appreciated. It shows respect for the local people and a willingness to adapt. Don't worry too much about perfect pronunciation—just say it with a big smile. Many people are likely to offer to be your teacher in exchange for a small fee. See below for the top phrases to master early on.

Top ten tips for communicating in English overseas

(Adapted from *WikiHow: How to Communicate with a Non Native English Speaker* edited by Invidia Cinelli, Bex, Jack Herrick, Krystle C., used with permission.)

1 **Speak clearly and pronounce your words correctly.** Exaggerated pronunciations will not help your listener and may cause more confusion. However, you may find that it helps to pronounce some words as the native speaker does. This will be especially true if the British pronunciation is very different from the native pronunciation.

2 **Recognise that people wrongly think that turning up the volume somehow creates instant understanding.** Avoid this common mistake (however, do not speak too quietly).

3 **Do not cover or hide your mouth because listeners will want to watch you as you pronounce your words.** This helps them figure out what you are saying in many cases.

4 **Do not use baby talk or incorrect English.** This does not make you easier to understand. It will confuse your listener and may give the wrong impression about your own level of competence.

5 **Avoid running words together** ('Do-ya wanna eat-a-pizza?'). One of the biggest challenges for listeners is knowing where one word ends and the next one begins. Give them a small pause between words if they seem to be struggling.

6 **As much as possible, avoid using filler and colloquialisms** ('um . . .', 'like . . .','Yeah, totally'). If your oral communication is filled with 'um', 'like', 'you know' or other fillers, comprehension is more difficult.

7 **If asked to repeat something, first repeat it as you said it the first time.** Then again. It could be that they simply didn't hear you. If your listener still doesn't understand, however, change a few key words in the sentence. It may be that they couldn't understand one or two of the words. Also repeat the whole sentence and not just the last couple of words. It's time consuming, but it helps prevent confusion.

8 **Consider the fact that your dialect may not be what the other person has learned in school.**

9 **Be explicit.** Say 'Yes' or 'No'. Do not say: 'Uh-huh' or 'Uh-uh'.

10 **Check understanding.** Your listener may nod but may not have understood. If understanding is important, e.g. in clinical situations, it is worth asking a couple of questions to check comprehension.

If your placement involves a lot of contact with local patients or staff (e.g. clinical or field work), then it is probably worth badgering a friend or colleague to start teaching you local terminology, such as common symptoms. Failing this, make sure a local speaker is around at all times—the local staff will quickly become your best friends in clinical situations!

Phrases you should master in the local language

(Adapted from *How to Learn Any Language*, http://how-to-learn-any-language.com, used with permission.)

Hello/Good morning/afternoon/ evening	Be aware of the exact time when you can say *Good morning* and so on. For example, in Spanish, after 12:00 people will correct you if you say *Good morning* instead of *Good afternoon*
Hi!	Find the most common informal greetings, as well as the latest 'in' greeting in the area you visit
My name is	Essential
Where are you from?	Also learn all the necessary explanations you need to answer this one
Are you married?	Also learn all the necessary explanations you need to answer this one
I'm learning your language but do not speak it very well	
Sorry Sir, I did not understand the word XXX. You see, I'm learning your beautiful language . . .	This one is to use when someone answered you rudely because you made a mistake or did not understand
How do you say that in (name of local language)?	A good tool to increase your vocabulary

Starting at work

"Steel yourself before going into work for the first time. There are likely to be a lot of shocks."

Emergency doctor, Guyana

The first few days at work can hold many surprises. No amount of experience, briefings or research will sufficiently prepare you for the madcap adrenaline rush of your first day at work in a new country, new health system and perhaps also a new language. The initial stark contrast between UK and overseas practice might even threaten to derail your settling-in process. If it all feels overwhelming or just too different, try to remember that it is still early on and that things will soon start to become more familiar.

Chapter 11 goes into much detail about some of the challenges of working overseas and the cultural differences that you may encounter. You may want to read this before you start work to know what you can expect and how you can prepare better. Below are some tips for those very first few days at work.

Be respectful of hierarchy

Acknowledgement of seniority and the local hierarchy can be more important in other health systems compared to the NHS. Pay courtesy calls at the start to your manager, the institution's director and whoever else you feel is relevant, so that they are aware of what you are doing and feel included in your work.

This will also allow you to introduce yourself to your colleagues, orient yourself and even attend a ward round or handover before the real thing.

Be ready for the lack of resources

Many health facilities will simply not have the drugs or equipment you consider essential back home. You may find that you can prescribe only one generic drug, when at home you were used to a selection of 20 or more. Diagnostic tests will be heavily rationed, and you will need to rely on your clinical judgement far more than in the UK. This can be difficult at first, and is likely to cause frustration throughout your stay; however, you will probably find that you quickly get used to working with the resources available.

Don't underestimate the workload

The NHS can be a very busy place, and most of its workers have a pretty heavy workload. However, in countries with few health workers and little preventative care, the workload can seem overwhelming even to NHS staff.

"I was put in charge of the paediatric ward, as well as two outpatient clinics a day and a cholera camp. This was when I was a relatively junior doctor. Added to this, my Pakistani colleague went on holiday for 2 weeks as soon I had arrived."

Paediatrician, Pakistan

Be aware of your colleagues' workload and try not to add to it unnecessarily.

"I would ask senior doctors coming to work here to be aware of your juniors' workload. Often this will be much heavier than what they expect. Don't write down long lists of jobs for each patient as there will always be more patients to be seen."

Malawian junior doctor, teaching hospital

Take your time to understand the local environment

> "The thing I find discouraging, borderline annoying, as an African, is people coming in and assuming they know the solution. What they should be doing is asking the questions."
>
> *Development Consultant, Côte d'Ivoire*

As an outsider to the culture and organisation, your first impressions may not accurately reflect the reality of the situation. A lack of in-depth understanding of the local norms and constraints may mean that what is sensible and logical to you, sits at odds with what is likely to work within the context. This may be because it is not relevant culturally or may not be a priority or equitable given the resources available. So before jumping in with ideas, making critical comments and suggesting changes, take time to research and really understand the local environment. Do make notes of your initial impressions though, as this is when differences will be most striking. Refer back to these after a few weeks or months and see if there is anything that you feel is still worth bringing up.

> "When I was put in charge of the paediatric department, I went round all the staff and asked what they would change if they could. I wrote all the responses down and tried to implement the most feasible ones over the course of the job."
>
> *Paediatrician, Pakistan*

Try to find a mentor. She/he may be another expat who has experience of the local working environment or a local who has an understanding of where you have come from. Your mentor can explain local nuances and the 'way things are done around here' at the beginning, and later play the vital role of a sounding board, helping to analyse and think through the correct way to move some of your work forward.

A degree of *innocence* can also work to your advantage, as it may help you to break through barriers and identify solutions which those working locally are constrained by. As a newcomer you can ask the complicated questions, which are more difficult to bring up further down the line. Questions along the lines of, 'I am just trying to understand why it is done this way?' or 'What was the reason for this decision?' Be curious, ask questions and you will be in a better position to understand the local context, the challenges that exist and also the possible opportunities.

Common problems in the first month

HOMESICKNESS/LONELINESS

Homesickness can be a symptom of culture shock; however, it is also a common feeling even in those well adjusted to their new culture.

You may feel a twinge of homesickness from time to time. This usually passes as you discover another exciting aspect of your host country or after a 'fix' of your home culture. Emails, cheaper overseas calls, Facebook and Skype have made staying in touch much easier, so you are much less likely now to spend weeks without any contact with home.

> "I stayed in a hostel in the town heavily visited by backpackers rather than in the area where my hospital was based. It was really nice to have ready access to internet cafes, cheap restaurants and the occasional beer or coffee."
>
> *Pharmacist, India*

After the first month (the end of the beginning)

If you have a long placement ahead of you, it is essential to make an effort to meet people early on. Not only will you have a more immersive and enjoyable experience for it, but you may also need their support when the going gets a little tough.

You may feel more reassured if you have made contact with at least a couple of other expats based near you before arriving. They will be able to provide an initial network of support and introduce you to others in the area.

However, it is very easy to fall into the trap of only making friends with other expats. They provide effortless company, and may share similar experiences and perspectives. But of course, if you choose to only do this, you will miss out. One of the joys of a longer placement is the chance to experience a different culture in depth—not simply skim along on the surface whilst maintaining your Western life. You may also find that some long-term expats can be quite cynical, with fixed ideas about the country, which may colour your first impressions. Be sure to make up your own mind.

> "When I first came to work in Africa, I decided I didn't want to hang around in expat ghettos and tried to only make local friends. While I did make one or two friends, our relationship was slightly limited. We come from such varied backgrounds that there were many things I couldn't discuss with them (laughing at cultural differences and misunderstandings, for example). So I now really appreciate my other foreigner friends, and feel like they are the only ones who I can share my situation with and who really understand me. Having a good balance of both is vital to understand the local perspective and maintain your sanity."
>
> *Health programme manager, Uganda*

Different levels of earnings can cause difficulties. Be sensitive to your friends' situations—their income is likely to support many people and not leave much for socialising. Paying for them may allow you to do things together—e.g. visiting a national park. (Of course, if you are doing your placement as a volunteer, you may find the difference in income is between you and other expats!)

> "I knew that my Namibian friends couldn't afford to eat out in restaurants, so for our social events I invited them all over to my house. I would buy the food and we would eat dinner together."
>
> *NHS manager, Namibia*

You may be asked for money from your new friends and, not infrequently, from complete strangers. This can be awkward and eventually frustrating. You may resent the image of rich foreigner, especially when you are volunteering. But in many cultures, giving to those in need is expected and is a central tenet of some faiths, such as Islam. People often support each other financially much more than we do in the West. Be clear, firm and consistent about what you can and cannot give—other expats can help you judge and deal with these situations.

Finally, see our tips for enlivening your social life. Friends will be a great source of support to you—so don't neglect this area in the mêlée of a new job.

Enliven your social life

- If you enjoy sport, **join a team**. You could check out whether there is a Hash House Harriers in your area. This is an international group centred around non-competitive running (or walking) and socialising, which exists around the world and groups meet once a week. They are generally a good mix of local people and expatriates, so it's a great way to meet new people, while exercising and exploring new areas (each week the *hash* run is held in a different area). For a worldwide directory of hash centres see *http://www.gotothehash.net*.
- **Rotary Clubs** exist all over the world as well and are an excellent way to network, make contacts and gain a greater understanding of the local environment.
- Find out if there is a local **cultural centre**, such as a local Institut Français, Goethe-Institut or Instituto Cervantes, which often put on an array of cultural activities.
- You may feel like you are missing out on good cinemas and films. If you have access to a projector and some good speakers, think about starting up **movie nights** at your house and get friends to invite other friends round.
- If you are in a remote area think about **travelling back to the city** every few weekends to get a dose of Western comforts.

➔

- If you are on your own, you may want to think about **sharing a house** with other foreigners. The houses are often large, with domestic help available (so no need to argue about who didn't do the washing up) and if your new flatmates have been living there for a while, they can provide a great introduction to your new city and a diverse range of friends. Many larger cities around the world have internet-based forums (e.g. Yahoo groups) or newsletters where housing may be advertised. Ask your contacts about this.
- If you are religious, join your local **place of worship**.

Common problems after the first month

Culture shock

Culture shock is a real phenomenon, and can lead to distressing symptoms which may curtail your trip overseas. It arises from the transition to an unfamiliar setting, where your value system and reference points are no longer valid. Culture shock does not always happen quickly or have one single cause. It often manifests after an initial honeymoon period, where you may feel that you are settling in well. It usually accumulates gradually from a series of events and experiences that constantly challenge your basic values and beliefs about what is 'right'.

Virtually everyone experiences some feelings of anxiety and uncertainty in a new culture. But for some people the required adjustment is very difficult and can overshadow their placement. If you find that you are experiencing any of the following symptoms, you may be suffering from culture shock:

- Excessive concern over cleanliness and health
- Feelings of helplessness and withdrawal
- Irritability
- Getting 'stuck' on one thing
- Excessive sleep
- Compulsive eating/drinking/weight gain
- Stereotyping host nationals
- Hostility towards host nationals

If so, try some of the strategies below to lessen the impact of culture shock. If you are struggling, do contact the person responsible for your welfare or placement. A period away from the environment and gradual re-introduction can often help with severe culture shock, as well as more support in your placement.

- Keep in touch with family and friends
- Remember what you would have done at home to relax and do something similar
- Do some familiar activities, especially the things you are good at
- Look for similarities between your culture and the new culture
- Ask questions when you are unsure about what to do or what is expected of you
- Try not to make judgements about others when they do things differently from what you are used to; remember, they are only different, not right or wrong
- Keep a journal or blog of your experiences—write down what you think and feel about what is happening to you. You could use this later to write articles on your experiences for other health workers considering time abroad.

(Adapted from University of South Australia, http://www.unisa.edu.au/ltu/ students/study/wellbeing/international/culture.asp, used with permission.)

Where to go for help
Your organisation

If your placement is through an organisation, then they are your primary contact point. There should be a regional or country co-ordinator who has primary responsibility for your welfare. Do flag up any problems (practical or personal) to them early, as they will usually have the local contacts to improve the situation.

"With VSO we had our own medical officer who gave us training on common health problems experienced by volunteers in Namibia which included a section on poisonous snakes and spiders and what to do in an emergency. It was reassuring to know that plans were in place if we did have a problem. We also had an evacuation plan in case our safety for any reason was compromised."

NHS manager, Namibia

Remember, nothing that you are experiencing is likely to be new to them. All these problems are extremely common, and you are not 'failing' or being a nuisance by wanting to sort it out.

Emergency health care

If you go with an organisation, do confirm the procedures for emergency healthcare when you arrive in-country. These should be robust, particularly if you are assigned to a remote area.

If you have arranged your own placement, you must check the availability of and arrangements for emergency healthcare. This is a tedious task when you have just arrived in an exciting new area, but essential. Make sure reliable systems are in place, as you won't have the luxury of time if something does happen.

See Chapter 9 for features of a comprehensive insurance policy. When you arrive, give someone at your placement (e.g. your supervisor or host) the company's emergency number and run through how to contact them—you probably won't be the one making this call if something goes wrong.

British embassy

The British Embassy in your host country has ultimate responsibility for your welfare as a foreign national. They can help in several kinds of emergencies. Register with the Embassy's LOCATE service online, as this will help you in case of emergency evacuation procedures (see Chapter 9). Below are five reasons why you should know your British Embassy's contact details overseas:

- If your passport is lost or stolen, they can issue you with a replacement one or, in some situations, an emergency travel document.
- If you're a victim of crime, they can help you get medical attention if you need it, contact your family and friends to let them know what has happened and give you a list of local lawyers and interpreters.
- If you have to be admitted to hospital, they can help you liaise with your insurance company or a medical evacuation company and they can contact your family and friends to let them know what has happened. They can also help if someone dies. They can't pay for your medical or repatriation bill though—which is why you need to have comprehensive travel insurance.
- If you run out of money, they can give you information on how to transfer money from the UK.
- If you're arrested abroad, call them as a priority. They can't get you out of prison, but they can contact your friends and family and provide lists of lawyers and interpreters. In some countries you're not entitled to call a lawyer, but you are legally entitled to call your nearest embassy wherever you are arrested.

© Crown Copyright 2011, Foreign and Commonweath Office.

And finally, do you know your embassy from your high commission? Your consulate from your mission office? British Embassy offices abroad are known by a bewildering variety of names, but this is worth getting to grips with as you're bound to come across them all:

- In Commonwealth countries they are called **high commissions** and located in the capital city.
- In other countries they are called **embassies**. These too are located in the capital city.
- **Consulates** are smaller offices in non-capital cities which offer assistance to British nationals.
- **Honorary consulates** are smaller versions of consulates in smaller cities and towns. Their prime task is to offer assistance to British nationals abroad.
- **Mission or delegation** is the name usually given to the offices attached to organisations like the UN and NATO.

Sometimes one office will cover several countries, so check the FCO website (http://www.fco.gov.uk).

Local police

The standards of local police forces vary by country and probably region. We have heard both good and bad experiences from fellow health workers. If you are in a situation where you need to interact with the local police, listen to people around you. Seek the advice of other expatriates and your organisation, including on the subject of bribes. In cases of theft, your insurance is likely to require a police report made within 24 hours of the incident. For more serious incidents such as assaults, your embassy is probably a safer first port of call.

Conclusion

This chapter has outlined some of the common problems you might face settling in to a new workplace and culture. Although this period can be difficult, be reassured that it will pass and you should soon be enjoying many of the daily wonders of living in a different country.

REFERENCES

Herxheimer A, Petrie KJ (2009). Melatonin for the prevention and treatment of jet lag. *Cochrane Database of Systematic Reviews* 2, Art. No. CD001520. DOI: 10.1002/14651858.CD001520.

National Travel Health Network and Centre (2010). *Health Information for Overseas Travel (the 'Yellow Book')*. London: Department of Health.

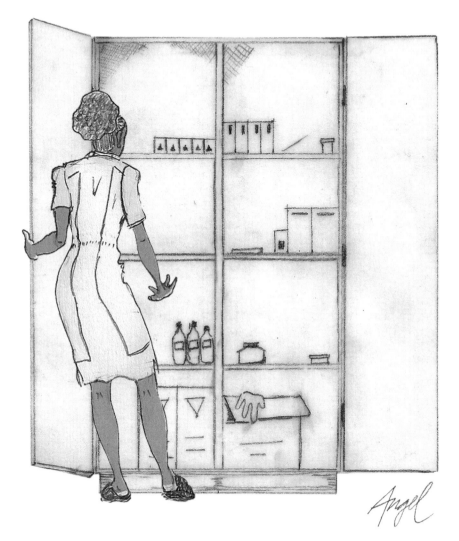

CHAPTER 11

At work

"The younger generation of doctors is often shocked by the conditions in LMIC. But for the older generation, many things are similar to what we encountered in the UK when we were newly qualified doctors. For example, the maternal death rate 50 years ago in the UK was only marginally lower than what it is in parts of Africa today. And the limited ability to provide treatment is also similar. Health systems, like democracies, take years to be built up."

Retired neonatologist and project manager

The aim of this chapter is to give you a snapshot of some of the situations that you are likely to encounter while working overseas. If you are reading this chapter while planning international work, it will help you to assess if and how you can work within these constraints. If you are already in post, it will help you analyse some of the issues in a bit more depth and how you can overcome them to work effectively.

The first section focuses on cross-cutting challenges, common to all types of international health work. Then we go on to look at the specifics of clinical practice, electives, humanitarian emergencies, teaching and training, research and project management in resource-poor settings. Chapter 13 then explores at how you can work within these constraints to bring about sustainable change.

Why do these challenges exist?

Weak or failing health systems, along with cultural differences, will manifest themselves in different ways: all will have an impact on your work.

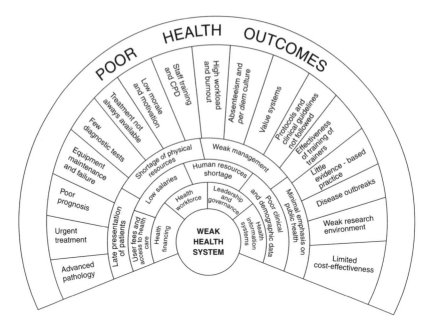

Figure 11.1 The influence of a weak health system on health outcomes and its impact on health workers.

Figure 11.1 illustrates some of the challenges of a weak health system, which ultimately result in poor health outcomes. These are discussed throughout this chapter. Not all will apply to every context, but we have cited those which are most frequently mentioned across a range of contexts. Specific challenges of individual contexts explored below are not covered within this diagram.

Common challenges

> "God, grant me the serenity
> To accept the things I cannot change;
> Courage to change the things I can;
> And wisdom to know the difference."
>
> *Reinhold Niebuhr*

Whether you are engaging in clinical work, teaching, researching or managing projects, you may come face to face with many of the following issues. They may initially be surprising and at times frustrating, but gradually you will adapt or learn to work within the limitations.

Working hours and time-keeping

Each culture has its own norms regarding working hours. Some countries may have a distinct lunch period where people go back to their families for a meal and most shops and businesses will close. There are often very practical reasons for them (e.g. not being out during the hottest part of the day, saving money by returning home for lunch) so it is usually easiest just to adapt to these new rhythms.

Low salaries, or no pay, may mean that staff are demotivated or need to take on two jobs to make ends meet. Time spent working can then be interpreted differently, as the following experience illustrates:

"The first day I arrived, one of the senior doctors left the busy department for 2 hours to go to the bank. I thought it was just the exception; however, the next day two of the other doctors left for the whole afternoon to go shopping. I was pretty shocked at this practice as there were many patients to be seen. However, I later realised that these doctors had not been paid by the government for 2 months. They were very demotivated and essentially working for free, so better they take a few hours out for themselves, rather than stop working completely."

Emergency doctor, Guyana

Time-keeping is another issue that many people comment on in particular countries. Your 2 p.m. may be the rest of the team's 3 p.m. Issues like this are often not just attributable to the individual, but to the system as a whole. If no one respects the start time of a meeting, the rational action is to arrive late to avoid waiting around. This can be very frustrating, and not just to you. If you are in a management position you might have an opportunity to change this aspect of the organisational structure.

"I would say, 'Everyone needs to come in for a meeting at 7 a.m. tomorrow'. And the first person would turn up at 7.20 and so on, so the meeting didn't start until 8. After a while I said, 'If you come late, you also have to work late'. Slowly the meetings are starting on time!"

Nurse, Rwanda

Shortage of health workers

The health worker crisis affecting much of the world was addressed in detail in Chapter 1. Lack of staff and specialists is likely to be most evident in a clinical setting, but will also affect other types of work. It can lead to several problems at work, which we will look at in turn.

HEAVY WORKLOAD

> "I would start at 7.00 in the morning, and often when I finished my shift there would be no one on the rota to replace me, so I would always end up staying an extra couple of hours."
>
> *Nurse, Somalia*

The NHS can be a very busy place, and most of its workers have a pretty heavy workload. However, in countries with few health workers and little preventative care, the workload can seem overwhelming even to NHS staff, with significantly less support and supervision available.

When you come to the end of your shift and there is no one to take over from you, you will face a difficult decision. Patients will not get attended if you leave, and you may end up staying long beyond your allocated hours.

BURNOUT

This can be a consequence of a sustained heavy workload or a result of excessive enthusiasm at the start of a placement. The many problems and injustices evident around you may impassion you to try and change the *status quo*. You may start a whirlwind of new services, or try to help your patients in much more than just their health needs. However, it is extremely important to know your limits.

If you experience over-exhaustion, you will not be helping yourself or the people you are working with. So learn your boundaries and give yourself time to recharge. Regular breaks away from the hospital are essential and offer valuable perspective.

Know the symptoms of burnout

Overworking and stress can cause burnout. It can be exacerbated by being in a new and difficult environment, especially if you feel you are failing to meet the constant demands. Burnout will reduce your energy and productivity, so it is important to recognise early signs which include:

- Depleted physical energy
- Emotional exhaustion
- Lowered immunity to illness
- Increasingly pessimistic outlook and problems may seem insurmountable

Those working in emergency contexts are usually given compulsory weeks of R&R or have time-limited assignments to decrease the chances of burnout. If you do not have these or are on a longer-term placement, make sure you arrange them yourself. Take yourself away to a restful place for the weekend, or a couple of weeks back home. Do not feel guilty: this is essential for your wellbeing.

ISOLATION

Coming from the NHS you will be used to being a member of a team, and having colleagues to talk to and bounce ideas off. Activities that may normally be carried out by a whole team at home can be the responsibility of a single person. If you are the only person with your skills, that responsibility becomes all yours.

Different practices and values

There will be many instances of differing clinical practice and cultural values. These may be considered as bad practice at home, or they may go against your professional values. Attitudes towards psychiatric illness, homosexuality, autonomy, privacy and confidentiality, and particular ethnic and religious groups may be very different to UK professional life.

> "On one of my first shifts, a boy who had drunk insecticide in a suicide attempt was brought in by his sister. He was very ill and needed medical attention; however, he was put in a corner cubicle by the staff and ignored. They felt that he had brought it on himself, and that their time was better spent on the many other 'blameless' patients.
>
> I found this difficult to see, although I could understand their frustration as they were extremely overworked. However, the sister was very distressed, and kept coming out of the cubicle to plead with staff to spend time with her brother."
>
> *Emergency doctor, Guyana*

Practices that may be taken as given in the UK, such as putting up screens for intimate examinations, may not occur in different contexts. At other times, a fatalistic attitude may mean that health staff are not willing to intervene.

Before you say anything, take a deep breath and consider the circumstances. What are the reasons behind this practice? Sometimes there are practical reasons, i.e. a shortage of screens or time, or people are used to addressing problems in the open. Side-step out of your own context and into that of your new environment. This will help you to start understanding the forces that dictate something to be done in that particular way.

This does not excuse or condone low standards, dangerous practice or discrimination. However, you will risk ill-feeling and resentment if you criticise without considering these contributory factors. As described later in Chapter 13, it may be better to lead by example.

Continuing professional development (CPD)

Keeping skills up to date and ensuring practice is evidence based is a continuous challenge in both low- and high-income countries. A lack of investment in this area can lead to inefficient and at times detrimental practices.

> "Every day, tens of thousands of children, women and men die needlessly for want of simple, low-cost interventions—interventions that are often already locally available. A major contributing factor is that the mother, family caregiver or health worker does not have access to the information and knowledge they need, when they need it, to make appropriate decisions and save lives."
>
> http://www.hifa2015.org

Access to information (such as a well-resourced library with access to up-to-date journals and an internet connection) is one challenge. Poor management and lack of reward for training also contribute, as may cultural differences such as an oral rather than written tradition of learning.

Do you know about HINARI and HIFA?

The **HINARI Access to Research Initiative** enables people in LMIC to access major biomedical and health journals online and free of charge. It is a joint initiative between the WHO and major publishers, making over 6,200 journal titles available to health organisations in 108 countries.
http://www.who.int/hinari

HIFA-2015 is working towards the goal of Healthcare Information for All by 2015. Its knowledge network has over 4,000 members representing 1,800 organisations in over 150 countries worldwide and is free. Members include health workers, publishers, librarians, information technologists, researchers, social scientists, journalists, policy-makers and others—interacting by email discussion forums, which include general and child health fora, and different language versions.
http://www.hifa2015.org

Encourage people to use these two excellent resources if they have access to the internet.

Some countries do require health professionals to undertake a minimum amount of CPD to stay accredited. And significant aid money has gone into improving evidence-based practice through workshops and trainings. However, this has its own issue: see the section on '*Per Diems*' at the end of this chapter.

> "I find that my colleagues like to discuss and debate at length, but no one has any real information, so they go in circles. I've never once seen people reading journals or appraising articles. Medicine works on facts and without them, how can we have an efficient health service?"
>
> *Nigerian doctor*

Governance, bureaucracy and regulation

> "We started up an NGO to raise funds in the UK and wanted to register it in our partner country, and do everything *by the book*. But the registration process was impossible; we had to get one paper from here, two from there, some signatures from people who were never in their office. A very drawn out process."
>
> *Project manager, Rwanda*

Systems and ways of doing things will differ. We often assimilate bureaucracy in our own countries, so the unfamiliar systems in LMIC often appear more complex. Sometimes you may feel that the bureaucracy decreases efficiency, while other areas will be relatively unregulated compared to the UK, possibly to the detriment of patient safety. Governance is an essential pillar of health systems, and more investment is needed in this area in many LMIC.

COUNTERFEIT MEDICINES

Counterfeit medicines are much more common in countries with weak regulatory systems. The WHO estimates that the incidence of counterfeit medicines is less than 1% in most Western countries, but much higher in LMIC.

Find out more
....
- WHO Factsheet on Counterfeit Medicines: *http://www.who.int/mediacentre/factsheets/fs275/en/index.html*

HIERARCHY

Hierarchy is an element of bureaucracy. While you may be used to an environment that encourages motivated individuals to take action; in many parts of the world, hierarchy, especially in relation to age and experience, takes precedence. This may result in the following (which are of course not unique to LMIC contexts):

- People at the top (e.g. hospital management) may be the most senior staff members or political appointments and not necessarily those with the best management and leadership skills. This may result in inefficiencies and dysfunction at top levels.

- If achievement is not rewarded, staff may have few incentives to perform well and may not be motivated to promote change.
- There may be little empowerment of staff at lower levels, which may mean little delegation from the top down. Managers may be involved in many of stages of decision making.
- As a young, qualified health professional, you may encounter some resistance or even antagonism from colleagues who are older but less qualified than you and who may see you as a threat.
- Women may find their authority is not well recognised by male counterparts in countries where female professionals are less common.

Unless you are coming into management or a position where you will have the authority to really promote change, you will have little opportunity to influence this permanently, and will therefore need to work within these constraints.

Make sure that you respect the hierarchy: getting those at the top on your side will be an advantage. Seek their advice and approval for any work that you are doing—and ask them what they think you should focus on and who else should be involved in this work. Be professional and maintain high standards at all times. If you gain their respect, it will make your life much easier: they are more likely to support your work and facilitate the required funding if it is available.

CORRUPTION AND BRIBERY

Corruption and bribery occur the world over, but it is the *in-your-face* aspect of bribery that is the most striking to people from resource-rich countries. This could be a parent openly offering you a bribe to accept their child into medical school or a patient offering a present to a doctor to get seen first. It is often seen as a way to overcome red tape and get things done more quickly in bureaucratic, inequitable or inefficient systems.

Transparency International's corruption perception index measures the perceived level of public-sector corruption in 180 countries and territories around the world.

In 2009, it found that out of the bottom 80 countries, the majority were low-income. Somalia, Afghanistan and Myanmar ranked as the three most corrupt countries.

http://www.transparency.org

You may be tempted to work within this system, in order to just get things done. Be aware that the UK Bribery and Corruption Act puts overseas transactions of this sort under scrutiny and essentially makes it as illegal for a British national to engage in corruption and bribery overseas as in the UK.

Clinical practice in a resource-poor setting

This next section focuses on challenges you may encounter when working in a clinical setting. Even if you are working in a different setting, it is useful to be aware of these as you will be more understanding of constraints faced by any clinical colleagues.

High mortality rate

"At the start of each day the doctor who'd been on for the night would report all the children who had died in the past 24 hours. It was a rare day when there weren't any and sometimes there would be as many as 10. On some days the number of children who died in the hospital in one night was greater than the whole number I saw during my 6 months as a paediatric senior house officer in the UK."

Palliative care doctor, Malawi

This is the stark reality in many LMIC. Death, whether from the effects of poverty, disease, injuries, resource shortages or illness, is part of daily life. Although many UK health professionals deal with death regularly, the sheer scale of mortality in LMIC can be overwhelming, especially in specialities like paediatrics.

What may also strike you as much as the death itself is the reaction of family members. Different cultures deal with death and grief in different ways, whether subdued or overtly. Local colleagues may also appear relatively indifferent; however, they have been working in this environment for far longer than you and will have become emotionally resilient. If you feel that it is affecting you and impairing your ability to work, recognise this and seek help from a mentor, project organiser or supervisor.

Late presentation

Some patients will present at hospital at the very last minute, when their condition has become so critical it is a case of life or death. Why, you ask yourself, did they not come here earlier?

User fees, traditional beliefs and access may all be the cause. In countries where patients need to pay for their healthcare, poverty will be the main reason. People may opt to wait, or try alternative treatments, only resorting to the health centre or hospital as a last option. To do so they may need to gather money, perhaps asking friends and relatives or selling personal items, to pay for the transport to hospital and the consultancy fees. Even in countries with universal and free healthcare, transport to the hospital may be a barrier.

In some countries up to 80% of the population depend on traditional healers (or 'witch doctors') for primary healthcare (WHO 2008). People turn to them partly through beliefs, but also due to availability. There will often be at least one traditional healer in even the smallest and remotest of villages, while the closest health centre may be many kilometres away. Other times people may not know that their condition is treatable. A typical example is epilepsy, which in many countries is associated with witchcraft or a curse on the family.

How might this affect you? Many diseases will be far more advanced before they present, and you are likely to see clinical signs that you have only read about before. Advanced pathology means the clinical diagnosis will be easier, but treatment may be more complex and outcomes usually worse.

Resource shortage

"You concentrate on diagnosing conditions you can treat, rather than rare diseases for which no treatment is available."

Neonatologist, Rwanda

Many health facilities will simply not have the drugs or equipment which you may consider essential back at home. This will mean that you need to adjust your ways of working and get used to the new system and the available resources. Equipment shortage or maintenance will affect your diagnostic ability and management options.

"I came to work in one of the four referral hospitals in Malawi for 2 years feeling that I had a lot to offer. I am a trained paediatrician, having completed my training 2 years previously. But in reality I found I couldn't be of much use as a specialist as I was unable to use many of the skills in the context. I am trained to work where there are resources and equipment. In Malawi I found a shortage of many of the equipment, drugs and diagnostics tests that I am used to working with on a daily basis. I only have five effective tests available to me: haemoglobin count; bedside blood glucose; cerebrospinal fluid microscopy; chest X-ray; and blood match. So clinically I feel handicapped. I know what the next step is, but I can't do it."

Paediatrician, VSO, Malawi

Diagnostic tests will probably be rationed, if they are available at all. You will therefore have to hone your clinical skills, as you will need to rely on these to make the diagnosis rather than investigations. Added complications may be that your patients may not be used to expressing their symptoms and you may not speak their language.

The WHO has produced a *Model List of Essential Medicines*. The core list presents a list of minimum medicine needs for a basic healthcare system, listing the most effective, safe and cost-effective medicines for priority conditions.

http://www.who.int/medicines/publications/essentialmedicines/en

Sometimes people also complain of smaller items of equipment going missing and so managers prefer to keep items under lock and key with restricted access. When salaries are low and there is burgeoning private healthcare industry, these items can fetch valuable amounts on the black market.

> "I was told that disposable gloves would be provided. However, when I got there, I found that these were in fact kept in a locked cupboard with the only key held by the senior sister. To get a pair of gloves before taking blood, for example, I had to ask her to come away from her patient and take me to the locked cupboard. I eventually gave up using gloves for minor procedures, but felt uncomfortable and would much rather have had my own supply."
>
> *Emergency doctor, Guyana*

Poor use of equipment

Ad hoc donations of equipment from well-wishers often supplement those procured by government. But it isn't uncommon to find valuable pieces of equipment gathering dust or locked away in a cupboard, unused. Why is this?

Lack of training for staff and a shortage of consumables and accessories all contribute to equipment lying idle. Sophisticated medical equipment can require specialised technicians to set up, maintain and repair. Staff also need training to know how to use new equipment for diagnosis or treatment.

Equipment may work for a short time, but when something goes wrong and cannot be easily repaired, it becomes redundant. Power fluctuation or black-outs may also cause damage to sensitive equipment. If reagents and consumables are difficult to procure, or a budget has not been set aside for this, the machinery also become obsolete once they run out.

If managed correctly, donations are important, but addressing systemic issues head on is an important sustainable achievement.

> "Quite often the light bulbs of our X-ray machines would burn out and need replacing. This is very cheap to replace, only about £0.50 or so, so you go ahead and buy it yourself, out of your own pocket, to be able to continue your work. But while it may not be a substantial cost to you, what will happen when you leave? The X-ray machine may go for weeks without working for lack of a bulb, and patients will be sent to the neighbouring hospital for an X-ray, at a substantial cost and risk to them. So while it is much more time consuming to procure it through the proper routes—you will be doing the system a favour. Look at distribution mechanisms, and see if you can do anything to improve or change these rather than doing things directly. Go through the correct routes, lobby, speak to people and share responsibilities."
>
> *Orthopaedic clinical surgeon, Malawi*

The response of many international visitors to equipment and drug shortages is to arrange donations. How can you ensure that these are appropriate and will be used efficiently? The 'Project Management' section below addresses good practice when organising equipment donations. Pharmacists Without Borders also publishes useful guidelines for drug donations (http://www.psfcanada.org).

Paying for healthcare

For those who have grown up with the concept of universal free healthcare embodied in the NHS, working in countries where patients must pay for healthcare can come as a shock. Once patients get to hospital, they may be refused entry unless they can pay an admission fee upfront (although many hospitals have charity systems for those most in need). For investigations and treatment, they may have to source further money from relatives or friends before this can go ahead, even when urgent.

If this is the case, be aware that all the tests or drugs that you are ordering for each patient will have to be paid at least in part by them. You may consider it all essential; however, each item may amount to a day's wage or more for them.

> "When I was asked to close up at the end of a patient's operation, I started suturing how I was taught in the UK: using plenty of suture and not cutting too close to the stitches.
>
> When the consultant looked over, he sternly told me that 'Il faut econo-miser!' (you must economise!). The patient had to pay for each new suture set we used in theatre, so the surgeons would use the minimum possible by tying tiny knots and wasting nothing."
>
> *Junior doctor, Madagascar*

WHAT CAN YOU DO?

Some of these challenges may seem insurmountable at first, but gradually you will adapt to the new way of working. The biggest challenge you may face is feeling out of your depth, due to being asked to engage in things that you feel are out of your competence. Know your limits. And make sure you read Chapter 12 on Getting the Most Out of it.

You may not always agree with the way some things are done, but it is important not to come in with your own firm ideas without first understanding the context. You can try to subtly change things (see Chapter 13 on Making an Impact), but be cautious about how you approach this.

Electives in a resource-poor environment

Going overseas on your elective is a very exciting prospect, especially whilst slogging away at undergraduate exams. However, if you are going to a resource-poor environment, then it's important to be aware of some potential situations which might arise.

Working beyond your competence

One of the great benefits of going on elective is being exposed to new conditions and procedures. Some students also return with reports of running outpatient clinics on their own or undertaking surgery with little guidance. The scarcity of other health workers and the often pressing need for healthcare can easily translate into feelings of cultural relativism, where 'having a go' seems preferable to nothing been done at all.

However, remember that your professional code applies as much overseas as it does in the UK. Outside of emergency situations (and sometimes even then), it is rarely preferable for you to undertake a procedure in which you are not competent than to wait for supervision to become available. If you don't have the skills required, say so politely but firmly.

The BMA suggests asking yourself the following questions if you are asked to do a procedure that you would not do at home:

- Why are you not allowed to do this procedure at home?
- Are you capable of performing it without suitable supervision?
- Are you putting your patient or yourself at risk?
- Would it be possible or practicable to ask for supervision without imposing excessive burdens on other health personnel?

(BMA 2009)

Cultural differences

If you are in training, and have only recently learned the 'right' way of doing something, it can be very tempting to point out the discrepancies with accepted practice back home. Don't offend senior colleagues who may be giving up their time to teach you: try to ascertain why these practices are in place before saying anything. Providing healthcare with little resources makes for clinicians with highly honed skills. Learn everything you can from them, and leave behind what feels wrong. You are likely to find several areas in which healthcare is provided in a better way than back in the UK.

"I was shadowing the colorectal team when they admitted a man who was having his anal warts surgically removed. He had caught them through homosexual sex, and the team treated him noticeably less sympathetically than their other patients.

I felt really uncomfortable with this, and went back to say some kind words to him later. Talking to a local colleague afterwards, it transpired that homosexuality is still very unaccepted in Madagascar. This didn't make it right, but it did make it more culturally understandable."

Junior doctor, Madagascar

Taking up time

Going overseas as an elective student is different to going once qualified. In the latter, you will be contributing your skills and experience. On elective, you are still not fully trained and your skills are, at best, in their infancy.

This is definitely not a reason to stay at home: the awareness and experiences you gain from elective will help you immensely in the multicultural world of the NHS and can spark off a lifelong love of international health. However, it is a reason to ensure you minimise the burden of hosting you, whilst still gaining from all the learning opportunities available.

With the scarcity of health workers in many LMIC, teaching time will be even more limited than at home. They have no responsibility to train you and any fees for elective students usually just cover administrative time. The learning needs of local students have to and should take precedence. Use your initiative to seek out good learning and teaching opportunities—don't expect to be directed. As in the UK, doing basic tasks to relieve the burden on local staff is likely to foster goodwill towards you and may free up time for teaching.

Finally, think very carefully about doing your elective where you will be using another language. Although it may seem the perfect opportunity to brush up, you may end up not learning much and draining considerable resources in time and translation needs if you do not speak at a high enough level. Refer to Chapter 6 for further guidance on languages.

Humanitarian relief

Humanitarian emergencies are intense and stressful situations. The pace is fast and you will have very little time to adjust to a new culture and norms before starting work. Disaster and danger bring even larger strains, and no one really knows how they will react until they get there. Although you will be part of a team, and their support is very important, you will need to be aware of and develop your own coping mechanisms. While many of the issues mentioned under clinical work will be applicable to emergency contexts, there are differences to working in an insecure versus secure environment.

Security

Security will play a massive part in your daily life whilst working in insecure environments. Organisations will constantly analyse and reassess the local conditions and risk factors. Rules may seem annoying and restrictive, but they are there to ensure your safety. Become familiar with security rules and protocols, safe and unsafe areas, protocols for engaging with international and local groups, and what to do in the event of a life-threatening situation, evacuation or kidnap.

> "While many organisations are good on security, there is always the potential for things to go wrong. I have friends who have been killed, and have seen security incidents threaten the whole of the project. It is really important to respect security rules."
>
> *Nurse, MSF*

Be sensitive to your new surroundings and gather as much information as you can about the context. If you feel unsure about anything, seek guidance from the project manager.

Health and safety

Your ability and time to look after your own health and hygiene is likely to be compromised. You will inevitably be much dirtier. Hand hygiene and all the principles of infection control that you have learnt will be as important as ever, of course, but so much harder to enforce. You may well have to work without masks or isolation rooms for infectious patients, e.g. TB, though you should *aim* to work in a well-ventilated room. This is often hard for people on their first foray into working in LMIC, but you will soon get used to maximising hygiene with limited resources.

You will undoubtedly receive briefings from your organisation, but Table 11.1 provides a useful summary.

Table 11.1 Health and safety measures in an emergency response

Protecting yourself from exposure to medical waste/ human remains	• Adhere to universal precautions • Protect your face from splashes of body fluids and faecal material by wearing glasses and a face shield (or cloth) that cover your eyes, nose and mouth • Use gloves to protect your hands from cuts and body fluids • Wash your hands with soap and water or an alcohol-based cleanser • Wear footwear that covers the entire foot and has thick soles to protect your feet • Dispose of clinical waste safely

➲

Protecting yourself from the heat	• Drink plenty of fluids and replace salt and minerals while working in hot weather • Wear appropriate clothing and sunscreen • Monitor the condition of your co-workers (for signs of confusion and even loss of consciousness) and have someone do the same for you • Take more breaks in extreme heat and humidity
Protecting yourself from the cold	• Wear appropriate clothing • Monitor the condition of your co-workers and have someone do the same for you • Make sure you don't allow yourself to become too cold
Ways to manage your stress	• Limit your working time to 12 hours per day • Rotate work assignments between high-stress and lower-stress functions • Take frequent short breaks • Keep objects of comfort with you (family photos, music, etc.) • Stay in touch with family and friends • Pair up with a colleague so that you can monitor each other's stress

Adapted from CDC: *Guidance for Relief Workers and Others Travelling to Haiti for Earthquake Response*, 23 October 2010. *http://wwwnc.cdc.gov/travel/content/news-announcements/relief-workers-haiti.aspx*.

Professional challenges

The difference between clinical work in resource-poor settings and humanitarian work may lie in the pace of the environment in which you are working. You are likely to be dealing with much higher numbers of people with acute conditions. You will not have much time to reflect and consult, and you will need to make split-second decisions and difficult choices.

On many occasions you will be treating diseases to which you have had little exposure, and you will need to develop skills that you may not have needed in your day-to-day job in the UK.

"In Congo, I got involved in delivering more babies in 2 months than in my last 2 years in the UK. Daily life must continue even in emergencies."

Paramedic, Doctors Worldwide

Not all humanitarian emergency work is about *putting out the fire*. Frenetic periods of activity may be followed by periods of relative inactivity when the workload is not as intense. You may be transitioning from the emergency to the rehabilitation phase.

Understanding cultural issues and local dynamics is imperative to be able to deliver care where needed and not exacerbate local biases. Cultural awareness is particularly important as you will need to identify and work with groups vulnerable due to their religion or ethnicity.

"The most rewarding experience was being able to apply what I had learnt during my diploma in tropical medicine at Liverpool to my work with refugees in Rwanda. I was able to convene a meeting at the refugee camp and identify among the refugees people who later became community health workers. Some of these people teachers, or had had a formal education, but not all. They contributed enormously to public health promotion around the refugee camp."

Doctor, Rwanda

Personal challenges

There will probably be several personal restrictions that will be imposed upon you for security reasons—from where and when you can go, to who your friends are. You may be spending 24/7 with the same people, living and working together, so it is vital that you get along as a team.

"Although I felt looked after, sometimes, after a while, it can feel a bit oppressive not to be allowed to leave the compound in the middle of the day on a Saturday. You just need to remember the local context and that, in the end, it is for your own benefit."

Paramedic, Doctors Worldwide

Living in areas of insecurity can cause acute stress. It can also wear you down through ongoing chronic stress. The loss of personal freedom, coping with different cultural norms or simple personality clashes all take their toll. Coping with minor stresses is a normal part of daily life, but it may lead people to engage in risky behaviour, such as heavy smoking, drinking, drug-taking or promiscuity. Try to be aware of your own reactions and how they may impact on your ability to do your job and being an effective member of the team.

Stress is sometimes experienced as post-traumatic stress. This is when you experience a traumatic event and the feelings generated at the time of the incident do not go away, but become more difficult and distressing. In most people, these will resolve eventually, but some individuals experience prolonged or worsening symptoms. Post-traumatic stress reactions are not abnormal or signs of weakness or inadequacy; they are normal responses to abnormal events. However, if symptoms are prolonged and start interfering with daily life, then it may be time to seek help.

Talk through any problems with team mates and speak to your project co-ordinator or line manager. Time out of the project (whether through R&R, annual or sick leave) can allow you space to rest and process your experiences. Don't be scared to seek professional medical help if needed. Early treatment is often better than hoping it will go away on its own.

Teaching and training in a resource-poor environment

Some of your time is likely to be devoted to teaching and training—whether it is running workshops, lectures or bedside teaching. To make this a success it is important to consider a number of issues.

Language

> "When I first started teaching during ward rounds I would get the most blank expressions from my students. They didn't interact with me, and I began to wonder whether they could actually understand what I was saying."
>
> *Neonatal nurse, Rwanda*

Your first issue will always be language—if people don't understand what you are saying your teaching sessions are futile. Speak slowly, simply, without using jargon or idioms (which are easily misinterpreted) and try to gauge what the level of understanding is. Even if they speak good English, it doesn't mean that they will be able to understand your strange accent and new expressions. If you keep slipping back into 'fast mode' write yourself a note to enunciate clearly and speak slowly. Chapter 10 gives some useful tips on adapting English so people can understand you.

If you need to teach in your second or third language, don't be too daunted. If it is also your student's second language, you may be at a similar level and able to understand each other better.

Resources

If you are preparing talks and lectures, think carefully what resources will be available to you. You are more likely to have blackboards and chalk than projectors and interactive whiteboards. Check with the course organisers what the students are used to and in what format they will expect the teaching.

> "I gave my lesson by talking and writing notes on the blackboard. However, the students were very disappointed with it. They were used to having PowerPoint presentations and then printing out the slides to use as revision notes."
>
> *GP, Malawi College of Medicine*

If you are using any sort of electrical technology make sure you have a contingency plan in case there is a power cut. And do provide all the materials along with your teaching, including diagrams and illustrations, not just summaries and bullet points like you might do at home. If books and internet resources are difficult to access, students will rely on your handout notes.

Methods

Consider your audience at all times. When introducing concepts, start at a basic level to ensure that everyone has the same understanding. Their previous studies may not have covered the topics to the same extent (or at all), so gauge prior knowledge at the outset and be prepared to cover the basics.

Teaching methods often vary significantly. While many countries are moving towards 'problem-based learning', the legacy of *chalk 'n' talk* often used at primary and secondary school can still be evident. See the pointers in Table 11.2 from Imperial College London to organise your teaching plan.

"In the UK I was used to problem-based learning, and interacting with the class, but at the beginning of my time teaching at a medical school in Uganda, my students didn't react well to it. 'Just tell us what we need to know,' they eventually told me. Blackboard lectures is what they have been used to; very didactic learning. But I didn't give up and eventually got them more involved in discussions and questioning what I told them."

Junior doctor, Uganda

Table 11.2 General teaching tips on basic teaching skills

Organising yourself	*When* am I teaching?—make sure you are prepared
	What am I teaching?—make sure you understand the aims and objectives of the session
	How shall I structure the lesson?—make a lesson plan
Basic teaching skills	*Setting the scene*—make sure that your students are comfortable and ready to start learning
	Being student centred—do you know what the students want to learn in each session?
	Assessing prior knowledge—check what the students know already

➲

Asking questions—keep your questions straightforward, but try to probe deeper levels of knowledge. Give the students enough time to answer

Checking understanding—make sure that the pitch and pace of the session is right

Using visual aids—it is worth taking time to find these, and using flip charts and overhead projectors wherever possible

Setting homework—vital to promote life-long learning, but check learning objectives and learning strategy are reasonable and ask students to present their work

Summarising and closing a session—don't give new information, and remind students about next week's topic

Source: Imperial College London (with permission).

"For my second trip to Sierra Leone, I spent 10 days teaching basic surgical skills to community health officers and junior doctors in northwest Sierra Leone. A consultation we did with our local partners had identified this as an area of great training need. Two surgical care practitioners and myself went with about £1,000 of surgical jigs [realistic plastic skin for practising suturing] donated by a local company ('Limbs and Things').

We had planned the training schedule before we left, so we were confident that we could achieve our learning objectives. However, on the day clinical staff from all around the country turned up and we ended up with double the number we expected! Other than that, it mostly went to plan. We did a knowledge test at the start and end of the course, and held a practical skills assessment on the last day. We also asked for global feedback on each session, so we could adapt the sessions as we went on.

Personally, I found the experience very stimulating. It allowed my colleagues to develop their teaching skills, which they don't have much opportunity to do in the UK. The next visit will be done by anaesthetic colleagues and will focus on perioperative care. We are planning to present our evaluation to the trust board before this to justify study leave for these visits."

Consultant surgeon, Sierra Leone

Training of trainers: how to make it effective

Training of trainers (ToT) is a popular concept within healthcare and it is also frequently used in development contexts. By passing skills on to local staff they are then able to continue training others in future. Or so goes the rhetoric.

But how effective is it? Although the ToT concept is considered cost effective, in many cases poor implementation and management of the process and an overemphasis on outputs (numbers trained) rather than outcomes (results of training) actually results in resource wastage. There are many cases where the desired 'cascade down' of expertise does not actually occur. In order to be most effective the ToT process should take into account the following issues:

- **Selection of trainers and trainees** is crucial as it can have a significant impact on the uptake of skills. Are those being trained the most appropriate and able people? Will they have the authority to train and advise others in future?
- **Incentives**. What will encourage those trained to change behaviour and train others? These need to be carefully analysed before training and can include financial and non-financial rewards, e.g. *per diems*, certificates, further career opportunities.
- **Context** is important for training to be transferable. For instance, carrying out a session in a state-of-the-art facility in a large city while expecting trainees to conduct their training in poorly resourced rural settings is a potential recipe for failure.

Conducting research in a resource-poor environment

Doing research overseas is a fantastic opportunity. Many people comment on the maturity and independence gained from working in such challenging settings. You may choose to do research overseas as part of a Masters or PhD, as a one-off project or as part of a longstanding research initiative. While many aspects of the research environment will be similar to the UK, there may be some peculiarities that you may not have anticipated. See also the section below on project management.

Supervision and support

The research community is likely to be small. You will have to work independently and may miss an exciting environment with lunchtime forums to discuss the latest papers in the *Lancet*.

If you are doing a PhD or research overseas for a long period of time, it is very useful to plan in regular trips back to the university with which you are registered for teaching, review of progress, exchange of ideas and access to high-speed internet and journals.

Equally it is important to choose your supervisors. You are likely to have to liaise with them on a regular basis, much more frequently than if you were in the UK with a dynamic team of colleagues. Choose someone who has the time to work with you, and if he/she is not based in your country, it is important that he/she has an understanding and direct experience of the context you are working with so that he/she can adequately support you.

Ethical approval

> "I believe it may be harder to get ethical approval in Uganda than in the UK. The Ugandan institutional review boards not only act to protect the study participants but also ensure that research being done in Uganda would be approved internationally. There is a concern locally that research takes place in Africa that would not be granted ethical approval in the West. Researchers should expect the process to be very rigorous."
>
> *Medical researcher, Uganda*

You will need ethical approval for any research involving patients or confidential data. Each country has its own process, but generally this will go through one level—the local Institutional Review Board—and in some cases a second governmental level. When you come to publish, most journals ask you to prove ethical approval.

This can take a long time to obtain and it is wise to apply at least several months in advance of commencing your research. Many countries will ask to get study information and consent forms translated into local languages as part of the ethics process. Find out what the exact process through your local contacts well in advance.

Jack of all trades

You are unlikely to have such a specialised team working with you during your research time overseas compared to the UK, so basic tasks will also be part of your responsibilities.

> "The research experience is very broad and I am involved at every step of the research process: protocol conception, ethical approval, community mobilisation, administration, financial accounting, all procurement, patient care and information feedback, sample collection and storage, laboratory assays, data collection, database cleaning, statistical analysis, and writing of grants and papers. At one point I employed 12 members of staff through my grant, and I believe in the UK a PhD student would not normally assume that level of management responsibility".
>
> *Medical researcher, Uganda*

This has positive and negatives sides, of course. You get to see the process as a whole, and gain significant generalist experience from this. On the negative side, many researchers who have spent long periods of time working overseas find it difficult returning to the increasingly specialist UK context.

Project management

Even if this isn't specifically your role, you may find yourself managing a project or a component of it while overseas. There are a few issues that you will need to take into consideration which may differ from your experiences of managing projects in the UK.

Logistics

For successful project management, you will have to think ahead, double-check all details and always have a contingency plan. Common problems include:

- **Power failures.** Do you have a generator at your main building/field site? Vaccines and blood samples can easily go to waste if power is off for long.
- **Roadworthy vehicles.** Finding suitable and affordable vehicles for long field trips over poor roads can be difficult in countries with no car production and expensive import duties. Make sure there is at least a spare tyre or two as these will have most likely been patched up previously.
- **Hiring staff.** Depending on the skills you require, hiring local staff can take longer than expected. Specialist skills are often in short supply, and you may need to allow extra time for training. Recruitment policies can be bureaucratic, and may delay your project. Be aware of nepotism and that your colleague may want to recruit his under-qualified niece for the post.

Per diems

When planning workshops or training sessions, you will need to think about whether you need to factor in *per diems* for participants. These are amounts of money given to participants to attend the workshop, essentially a sitting allowance. They are usually given in addition to transport and accommodation costs.

Per diems?
....

In the early days, the aid agencies, eager to attract all the best people to attend their training, started rewarding people's attendance in *per diem* payments. In many countries, especially sub-Saharan Africa, this is now firmly engrained in the system. Participants may not turn up to training sessions if it does not offer a daily allowance. So at times it may seem that the best people are always off on some training or another and never at work. Three or four days of *per diems* may amount to their total monthly salary, so on very low wages it is an important source of income for many.

Per diems can have negative repercussions, including the wrong people attending training courses—merely to collect them.

If you don't plan to give out *per diems*, you must state this clearly when participants are invited. This ensures that you will get the most motivated workers attending, but it can be hard to enforce. People may feel they are being discriminated against, or that organisers are being corrupt by not distributing the *per diems* allocated. When planning budgets, check what the local situation is. If you do plan to pay *per diems*, see what the government going rates are, which usually vary from grade to grade.

Transport refunds, overnight accommodation and food will need to be included regardless. Facilitators and speakers will also expect to be paid, and have transport and accommodation provided for them, so factor this in too.

Timing and communication

> "We had organised a workshop weeks in advance, but I was furious when I arrived and found out my colleague coordinating the attendees only rang them up that day to say 'come tomorrow'. I was worried no one would be able to attend at such short notice. But most people turned up. It seems to be the way things are done here, although I am not sure it's the most efficient way to work. I still think most people appreciate being told at least 2 weeks in advance, but at least it is still possible to do things last minute."
>
> *Project manager, Ghana*

Things may happen on different time scales compared to what you are used to. Some things may happen much quicker, while other, seemingly simple things will take longer. Factor these in when planning the time scales of any project, and be prepared for last-minute changes of plans when some key participant is urgently called away on important business.

While email is becoming more and more popular as a method of communication, it is best not to rely completely on it. Mobile technology has really taken off and is often the preferred method of communication. So much so that you shouldn't be surprised with the different etiquette around mobile phones—people may answer their phones in the middle of a meeting or workshop, when you would deem it totally inappropriate to do so.

> "When we delivered week-long training to communities out in the rural areas we would also provide the food for the week. As there were no refrigerators, we would take two live goats with us as that was the only way we could provide fresh meat!
>
> Communications with our volunteers could not be done by email or even telephone. When we needed to contact members in the rural communities, we would use the bush radio. This was a local community radio station that would broadcast notices. It always amazed me how efficient this would be as everyone would turn up to meetings publicised in this way!"
>
> *NHS manager, Namibia*

Procurement

If you are procuring goods and equipment from outside the country, remember that transport can be very costly and factor in customs fees and duty clearance on arrival as well. What about maintenance of equipment? It may be more cost-effective to procure through a local company which can also be involved in maintenance.

Before ordering, requesting a donation or going about repairing a piece of local equipment, think about installation, usage and upkeep. Locally sourced equipment with companies that have in-country representation is more likely to have technicians on hand to repair it when it breaks down. You will need to consider the following:

- Is it a necessary, relevant and cost-effective piece of equipment?
- Do you have a plan for the proper management of donated equipment?
- Do staff have the skills to use and maintain the equipment?
- What training might they need?
- How much does transport, shipping and local customs clearance cost?
- Is there a continuous supply of any necessary consumable or reagents?
- Can consumables be sourced locally and within budget?
- Who will be in charge of maintaining the equipment and repairing it when it breaks down?
- Will you need any electrical equipment to protect it from power fluctuation or different currencies? Has a budget been set aside for this?
- How will the effectiveness of the piece of equipment be evaluated?

The onus is on both the donor and the receiving health organisation. All too often a recipient will accept items with open arms, often without putting adequate thought into the running and maintenance costs. Try to encourage good practice in relation to any equipment donations.

Find out more

The WHO has produced guidelines on equipment donations:

- *Guidelines for Heath Care Equipment Donations*. WHO, 2000. *http://www.who.int/hac/techguidance/pht/1_equipment%20donationbuletin82who.pdf*

Other good resources include:

- *Beyond Good Intentions: Lessons on Equipment Donation from an African Hospital*. Stephen Howie *et al.*, 2008.
  http://www.who.int/bulletin/volumes/86/1/07–042994.pdf
- *Guidelines on Medical Equipment Donation. The Pharmaceutical Programme—World Council of Churches (WCC) and Community Initiatives Support Services.*
  http://www.drugdonations.org/eng/richtlijnen/eng_guidelinesequipmentdon.pdf

Conclusion

This chapter has highlighted some of the challenges you are likely to encounter on a daily basis, why they may occur and how you can work within these constraints. Chapter 12 looks at how you can keep your professional development on track whilst working overseas.

REFERENCES

British Medical Association (2009). *Ethics and Medical Electives in Resource-Poor Countries: A Toolkit*. London: BMA.

World Health Organization (2008). *Traditional Medicine*. Fact Sheet N134, December 2008. http://www.who.int/mediacentre/factsheets/fs134/en/.

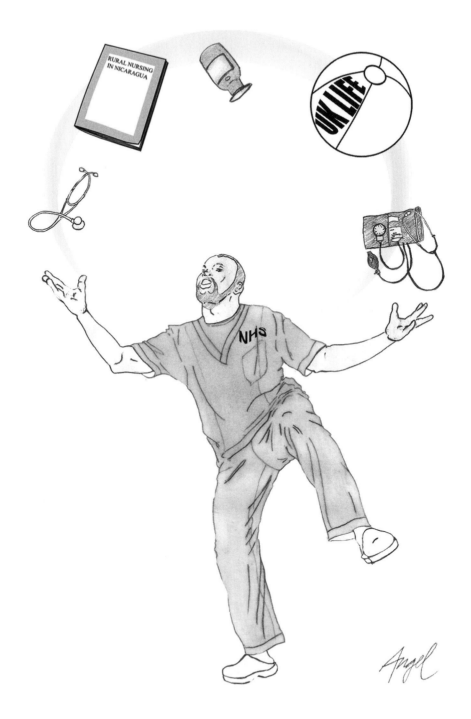

CHAPTER 12

Getting the most out of it

Iinternational work is exciting and full of opportunities. But not many of these are associated with enhancing one's career back home. In fact, the one stumbling block preventing many people from taking the leap into international work is the concern of how it may affect their career after their return.

With the right planning you can make an international post work in your favour. Keep an eye out for the possibilities and another for evidence to demonstrate the competencies you have gained. Chapter 3 looked at the rewards and challenges of this type of work. Here, we look at how you can maximise the rewards and reduce the challenges.

The chapter is divided into two sections. The first part looks at how you can ensure your overseas work does not negatively impact on your UK career or, even better, how it can positively influence it. The second part of the chapter is targeted at those people who want to stay in the field of international health, be it as a full-time career or combined with NHS work.

Maintain (and enhance) your UK career whilst overseas

Find a mentor or educational supervisor

You may be surprised to find that you change from being a junior staff member in the UK to a highly qualified and relatively senior person when overseas. This often translates into little support and supervision. For your own motivation and personal development it is advisable to find a suitable mentor or supervisor, especially on long-term placements.

> "I liaised with my supervisors (one in the US, one in the UK) on a weekly basis during my PhD in Uganda and sought their support for both technical and logistical issues. I had no one else locally whom I could interact at that level and bounce ideas off."
>
> *Medical researcher and oncologist, Uganda*

You may even want to find two mentors: an incountry mentor who can help you with the local practice and context—if there is no one at your workplace who can fulfil this role, look to the surrounding larger organisations—and a second one back in the UK who can update you with developments and training back home and support on other issues. When choosing a mentor or supervisor, it is important to do so carefully. Select someone who:

- Has the time to devote to you, perhaps an hour a week or so, with the possibility of field visits if relevant
- You are able to communicate easily (and cheaply) with, for example using Skype, email or cheap phone calls
- Has an understanding of the context you are working in (particularly relevant for your UK-based mentor), so that he/she understands the challenges you are facing

If you are a doctor in training and taking the time as OOPT (see Chapter 4), then you usually need to have an accredited trainer in your overseas organisation. This means that he/she is a member of your Royal College and has done courses on training. He/she will be able to sign off competencies for your training portfolio. Even if you are not taking it as OOPT, it is worth finding someone locally who can provide you with educational support.

> "Although I didn't have a UK mentor, I did have a local mentor. He didn't have the time to supervise me constantly, but he was happy for us to have a joint clinic once a week. This gave me the opportunity to learn a lot about local practice and discuss any difficult cases that I had come across. He also made important introductions to other health professionals and eased me through the process of getting officially approved to practise in that country."
>
> *Junior doctor, Bolivia*

However, remember that your mentor or supervisor can only provide limited support, so make sure you have the skills and competency at the outset to adequately approach your work.

Identify the experience and skills you want to gain

Think about your medium-term career goals and refer back to the skills diagram in Chapter 3 (Figure 3.2). What competencies would you like to gain? For example, would you like to gain some more teaching experience? Do you have an interest in management? Might your expertise be of use in policy-making or developing protocols?

Explore avenues to gain these skills. Your time abroad will present you with a range of opportunities which you can tailor towards your personal and professional development. Of course, you'll need to make sure that you are fitting into existing plans, rather than creating parallel projects around your specific areas of interest (see Chapter 13).

> "During my year in Bolivia [as well as running a mobile clinic]. I also became heavily involved in developing a plan for long-term care of patients with type 2 diabetes in the department of Oruro. This was a huge task and I certainly never expected to be involved in public health planning on a departmental level."
>
> *Junior doctor, Bolivia*

Keep a portfolio

Many people, especially those with no international experience themselves, may view your time overseas as a jolly, not to be taken seriously. You can counter this attitude by providing evidence for everything you have done during your time overseas. Keep a folder with details of all the practical and theoretical experience that you have gained overseas (see box). This should be familiar to most health professionals, especially if you already have to demonstrate CPD for registration purposes.

What to put in your portfolio

- Log book of practical procedures/operations
- Short summaries of interesting cases and cases you have learnt from (especially those you would not have had exposure to in the UK)
- Supervisor's report
- Annual appraisal
- Publications
- Audits
- Copy of rota
- Certificates of attendance on courses and at conferences
- Teaching plans/evaluations
- Agendas for management meetings where you presented

➲

- Thank you letters from patients and juniors
- Photos for reports/presentations/blogs
- Local/national/international news clippings about your work or showing the need for it

If you have been overseas for a while, expect to return with quite a hefty tome. This is essentially the evidence of your CPD whilst overseas, which you will need for registration, revalidation and interview purposes.

Keeping notes at the beginning, when you are at your most perceptive, will be a good reminder of your initial impressions and help you to talk enthusiastically about it later. Striking differences in case-mix, practice and health systems will quickly become normal to you, so it is useful to have that reminder. This can produce the superlatives about your situation which will help you to 'sell' your experiences in applications or interviews back home.

Have an annual appraisal

If you are going to be abroad for more than 1 year, ask your educational supervisor for an annual appraisal. For many health professionals, this is needed for registration. For doctors who are OOP, this needs to be submitted to your deanery to maintain your national training number. Appraisals can be more than just rubber-stamping though: a good appraisal will allow you to review your work, identify any learning needs and even develop a personal development plan (see next section).

Keep your knowledge up-to-date

If you plan to be away for a long period of time, decide how you will stay up-to-date with the latest developments in your field. If you have reliable access to the internet, you can do this via online journal subscriptions—if you do not have an Athens password (note that most NHS staff are eligible for an Athens account), you may be able to access journals through HINARI (see Chapter 11). Online discussion forums (such as http://www.doctors.net.uk) and any professional email groups are another good way to keep up with debates and controversies within your field.

If hard copy is your preference, subscribe to some journals and get them sent out to you, or ask colleagues in the UK to send their back copies to you in a bundle. Alternatively, download interesting articles during a trip back home or to the main city, and save these on a memory stick to read at your leisure. If you are in larger institutions you may find some journals there too.

It is also a good idea to schedule in (and budget for) international conferences at least once a year to keep abreast with the latest developments. As described above, keep evidence of everything you have done for your return home.

Cultivate your contacts in the UK

Make sure you don't fall 'out of the loop' while you are overseas as this can make finding a job on your return much harder. This is particularly relevant to those in management positions where contacts can play a pivotal role in recruitment.

Do make an effort to stay in contact with old colleagues and key contacts. A good way to do this is to attend important professional meetings in the UK (such as your Royal College or professional association's annual meeting) where you can network with many contacts in one place.

You might want to keep contacts up-to-date with your work via a blog or newsletter. Make them realise that you have not just got itchy feet and disappeared on a gap year, but instead you are doing serious work and have as much (if not more) responsibility than you did in the UK.

> "I went to Tanzania to work with the Agha Khan Foundation for 1 year. When I returned, I got a job straight away, mostly thanks to the contacts that I had maintained while I had been away. My overseas experience was seen as a strength of character and rewarded."
>
> *NHS manager, Tanzania*

Publish your work

Having your experiences from your work overseas published is an excellent way to gain credibility and recognition for this time. You don't need to be involved in research to do this, as case reports, articles about your experiences and policy work will all be of interest. Chapter 13 will help you think about how to evaluate the impact of your work, which could also be the subject of a publication. Don't despair if it doesn't get into a high-impact journal: articles in organisational newsletters and policy bulletins can be put on your CV and will disseminate your learning just as well. Even better, work in collaboration with local colleagues to help them to gain experience and recognition too (see Chapter 13).

Journals with a focus on international or tropical health:

- *Tropical Doctor*
- *East African Medical Journal*
- *Tropical Medicine and International Health*
- *Human Resources for Health*
- *Health Policy & Planning*
- *Rural and Remote Health Journal*
- *The Lancet*
- *Alma Mata Journal of Global Health*

Plan your re-entry early

Unless you can afford some time off to look for jobs when you return to the UK, it is advisable to start looking at what is available before you leave. Having a job or interviews to come back to will also help you to re-adjust to life in the UK.

Plan time to look for jobs online (visit http://www.jobs.nhs.uk and http://www.mmc. nhs.uk for post-graduate medical training), use your contacts to find out about jobs, and remember that interviews can take place 6 months before the advertised start date.

Elective students

For medical students, electives can often fall in the same period as Medical Training Application Service (MTAS) applications. If you're away during the deadline, plan ahead so you have a relatively stress-free experience.
Make sure you:
- Get hold of last year's application form so you have an idea of the questions. They are unlikely to change that much, so plan out basic answers before you go away
- Try to plan your time so that you are in a major city or town with reliable internet access during the period of the online application
- Ask a friend to send you a copy of the questions as soon as the online application is open—so you can get started even if your log-in initially fails
- Upload your application at least a few days before the final deadline. The website has been known to crash in the final 24 hours, and you definitely don't want to be calling UK helplines on your elective

---

Make your time overseas work for you

Many people's first foray into international work generally ignites a lifelong passion. So prepare to be hooked—if you are not already.

If you intend to have a lifelong involvement in international health, be it as a full-time career or combined with a UK career, your time overseas will present you with many opportunities to work towards this goal. This section gives you some ideas on how to maximise these to your long-term advantage.

Build up local contacts

Colleagues, managers, district officials, even people within the ministry or the Minister of Health him/herself—these are all people you may come into contact with. It will take time to build up their trust and for a friendship to develop. But when it does, it may serve you well.

If you want to stay involved in international work, maintaining these contacts is essential. People prefer to use a reputable contact who they know and can trust, so you never know what may emerge years down the line.

"At the beginning I found people courteous, and very polite, but perhaps understandably somewhat cautious. After a few trips back and efforts to understand more fully the local needs and priorities, people began to understand more clearly my longer-term objective to support their programmes of medical education. That is when we started to build real friendships and plan our joint project. The Dean and I secured external funding to establish a consortium of West African medical schools and develop a teaching partnership. My colleagues and I now return several times a year to support their teaching and examining. You can only do this once trust between those involved in the project has developed."

Professor of medicine, Nigeria

However, the movers and shakers are not just people in government. There will often be a network of international NGOs locally, which are worth getting to know whilst you are there. They could provide opportunities for you in future, as many have long-term projects and/or are involved in policy-making and planning. See also the principles of alignment and harmonisation in Chapter 13.

Get informed

The best place to learn about the global health jigsaw is in the field. The more you read and speak to people, the more you will understand how all the pieces fit together and where future opportunities may lie for you. Living overseas, you will meet and socialise with health professionals, policy-makers, NGOs, international health consultants and journalists who may have worked and lived in the area for years. Their insights are often fascinating. Do take time to listen and look outside of your niche area.

Learn the language

If you want to continue working internationally, speaking languages will be a huge advantage and will give an edge over other candidates in competitive jobs. It is likely that your patients will speak an obscure local dialect. Do learn this if you have developed a passion for the region and intend to continue working there. Alternatively, opt for a more widely spoken languages for longer-term investment—Swahili, Arabic, French, and Spanish are particularly useful.

Evaluate your impact

If you have done good work and made an impact, you will need to show the evidence. Donors are much more interested in funding further work if previous phases have been properly evaluated to show evidence of learning and success. This doesn't need to be formal research (although it may lead on to this). Simple audits or quality improvement reports can help to highlight your impact. Do try to factor this in right at the start of your work as it will help make the task much easier. There's more on this in the section on Monitoring and Evaluation in Chapter 13.

Draw up a personal development plan

If you want to stay involved in international health work in future, look at how you can build up your skills and experience to be more marketable in the field. Personal development plans (PDP) are widely used both in the NHS and in business. They aim to help you reflect on your achievements and learning to date, and plan for your continued professional and career development. A PDP provides a framework for prioritising skills that need to be developed, planning the necessary courses or activities, monitoring progress towards these goals, and evaluating the outcome at a set date, e.g. in 1 year's time. If you don't have one, develop one for the length of your placement.

Think about what type of international work you would like to get involved with, what skills are required by recruiting organisations (see Chapter 7) and how you can gain these (see Appendix 3). Ask your mentor or someone senior in international health to review your PDP to see if it is on-track.

Identify opportunities for continued involvement

If you want to stay involved in international work, try to identify opportunities where you and colleagues back in the UK can provide support. The best time to do this is whilst on the ground. Where are the gaps? Do they need mentors or supervisors for staff? If a regular programme of training is needed, would it be best to set up a Health Link? Are there opportunities for continued collaborative research? See Chapter 15.

And finally

Look after yourself

In order to get the most out of your time overseas, it is important that you keep yourself in good mental and physical condition. Burnout, psychological problems and culture shock are all real possibilities. It is also easy to neglect your diet, sleep and exercise routine when out of your normal surroundings. If you experience over-exhaustion, you will not be helping yourself or the people you are working with. Learn your boundaries and give yourself time to recharge. If you feel that something is affecting your work, identify what it is and seek help, whether this is a discussion with your mentor or a weekend away to recharge your batteries.

Take opportunities to travel and explore

While you will be overseas for work, it is also a great opportunity to travel and explore the region in your time off (your ability to do this will depend of course on local security). Do remember though that road traffic accidents are one of the biggest killers of expatriates abroad, so follow our tips in Chapter 9 to minimise your risk. Overseas work can be very intense, so enjoy your time off.

Tie up loose ends

As with any job, it's easier to tie up loose ends before you leave. Get any important signatures or references now, finish off any audits and work out the contributorships to any research projects whilst everyone is in the same room. Don't think 'I'll just email them when I'm back in the UK'—memories fade fast, especially when the other person is now in a different country.

Conclusion

You now know the best ways to make your time overseas work for you. The next chapter will look at how you can maximise your impact from a different perspective: your organisation and your host.

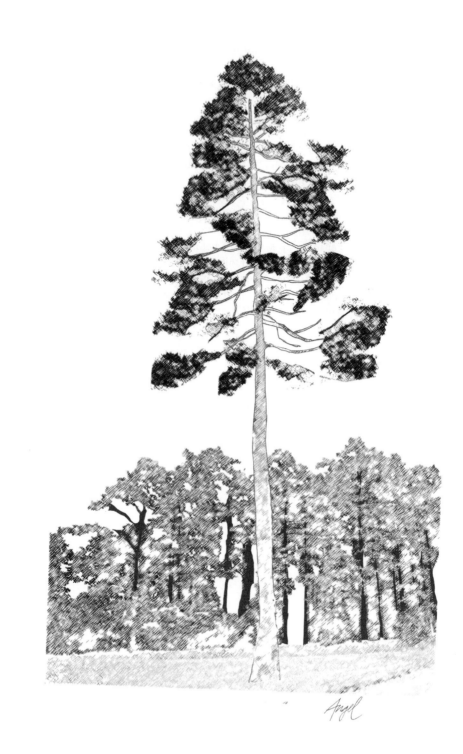

CHAPTER 13

Making an impact

> "Vision without action is merely dreaming.
> Action without vision is simply passing the time.
> But vision with action can change the world."
>
> *Nelson Mandela*

You now know how to get the most out of your time overseas. But how can you extend this to the communities and organisations you work for? This chapter will help to get you thinking about how you can maximise the impact of your work overseas.

The *first* section explores small things that can have a big impact. This part is relevant to everyone, whether you are an elective student doing limited hands-on work or a researcher, clinician or manager.

If bringing about lasting changes is a specific aim of your time overseas, the *second* part of this chapter introduces some useful principles for international engagement and effective ways to produce sustainable change.

The *third* and final section looks at how to measure and understand the impact that you are having. This will help you to learn from and modify your work, and will be important for your hosts, organisation and any donors who have helped to support your time overseas.

Sustainability

If you are applying for any sort of project funding or grant, you will probably be asked how your work will be sustainable (beyond the end of the funding/your time overseas). This is often demonstrated through teaching and 'building local capacity' (see below).

"We are under pressure to show how our work is sustainable, so my clinical work is done under the pretence of teaching, rather than gap filling. But there is a big gap: I am one of two neurologists in this country. When there are many patients to see, I would prefer just to work as a clinician, treating my patients, as I do in my own country."

Neurologist, Rwanda

'Sustainable development' was a concept first used in relation to the environment, meaning development that 'meets the needs of the present without compromising the ability of future generations to meet their own needs' (World Commission on Environment and Development 1987). Sustainability has now become a very broad term essentially meaning 'the ability to endure over time'. This is more likely if 'initiatives [are] supported by long-term commitment from all parties involved. If the initiative is only undertaken by an individual, however motivated, with little institutional buy-in, the activities are likely to fall by the wayside when the individual moves on' (Department of Health 2010). If you are working towards lasting change, it is vital to think about sustainability.

Small things can make a big difference

"Everyone who goes to work overseas, with their egos, wants to start something up, make a change."

Doctor, India

During your time overseas, you will be interacting with a wide range of people who will be continuing their work on the ground after your departure. How can you motivate and influence others to promote change that will remain after you leave?

Personal relationships are very important, and the capacity to inspire, motivate and encourage others is a key skill. In an environment with few health workers, senior specialist support is often minimal. Coming from a different environment, you can help promote a two-way exchange of ideas, which is a key driver of development.

Lead by example

> "When we are medical students we learn the theory of how things should be done correctly. But when we qualify, perhaps we become lazy, or adopt some of the bad practices of our senior colleagues. So it is good when we have visiting doctors from other countries to come to work with us. We observe how systematic their note taking is, how they do examinations, how they present histories, and we like to learn from them."
>
> *Rwandan junior doctor, teaching hospital*

Remember that we suggested in Chapter 10 to take time to understand the local environment before criticising the system or trying to change things. Where you do feel practice can be improved, don't be openly critical as this can create antagonism and resentment. Instead, lead by example. By demonstrating good practice and alternative, perhaps better ways of doing things you will make colleagues aware that other ways are possible. If they see the benefit in doing it your way, they will want to learn from you.

> "Although I don't think criticising other people's practice is helpful, there is no reason why you can't set a quiet example. I made a point of telling all my patients their diagnoses and asking if they had any questions. I would also move female patients to a private cubicle if they needed a vaginal examination. This approach isn't confrontational, and you never know who you are influencing around you."
>
> *Emergency doctor, Guyana*

Encourage success and enthusiasm

One of the main reasons cited for health worker migration is access to opportunities for learning, training and career progression (Awases *et al*. 2004; Crisp 2010). For those who are motivated, there may be few incentives: good work is not always rewarded and on the flipside poor practice is not always picked up either.

As Chapters 1 and 11 have described, health workers in low-income countries work in very difficult conditions. Trying to live off a poor or non-existent salary, working with old or broken equipment, being unable to provide treatment to patients because there are no supplies, and going for months on end without any senior support would break most people's morale. The fact that there are still functioning health systems in most countries is a testament to the determination and professionalism of their health workers.

Do not be surprised if sometimes your local colleagues lack enthusiasm or motivation. Your challenge is to renew their drive by inspiring them and showing them that success is possible. Identify those who you can encourage in their work, and who could go on to become drivers of change themselves. If they feel supported, they are more likely to go on to achieve more. Be friendly and approachable and give them a platform to improve themselves.

"I helped to run a nurse development programme in Gondar (as part of a hospital—hospital Health Link). At the end of the workshop, each nurse identified key things to go away and put into practice. The nurses left the workshop with good intentions, but pressures back at work meant that many of them did not turn their plans into action, as happens frequently in the UK.

One nurse, however, did. Quietly and singlehandedly she managed to use what she had learnt in the workshop to make a huge change in her hospital's laundry facilities, with the resulting improvement in infection control.

With encouragement, she had demonstrated that she was a person who could bring about change, and someone who could be relied upon in future to put plans into action."

Nurse consultant, Ethiopia

You can provide this support in various ways. However, be aware that sometimes your support can be misunderstood as excessive micromanagement by local staff, or a case of the 'foreigner thinking he/she is better than us', so tread carefully.

If you are **senior** to them:

- Try to provide extra on-the-job training and explore the possibility and need for formal training or workshops.
- Provide mentorship on a long-term basis, either in person or remotely after you return home. You could discuss specific cases or journal articles, work towards joint publications or give advice on career progression,
- Give direction to resources such as online training and funding opportunities for training, and encourage them to apply.

If you are the **same level or junior**:

- Set up regular opportunities for joint learning, e.g. grand rounds or journal clubs.
- Share books and journals which cover their areas of interest. Or encourage them to get access to online materials such as HINARI (see Chapter 11).
- Give help to link up with more senior colleagues back at home who could provide mentoring.

- Engage in joint initiatives that could help build confidence, such as a joint research project or audit.
- Learn from them, as this is a great opportunity for mutual exchange of ideas.

"I first visited in Uganda in 1995 as a visiting lecturer in psychiatry, where I met a small but excellent group of qualified psychiatrists keen to develop ideas and exchanges. Their research output and publications were meagre. This was due to many factors including access to grants and lack of experience, confidence and access to international journals. Together with a Ugandan colleague who shared an interest in research we started writing joint papers for publication. We initially targeted professional journals rather than peer-reviewed publications, for example giving accounts of psychiatry and practice in East Africa. At first I led the process, doing the bulk of the writing and liaison with editors, while my Ugandan colleague contributed facts and figures. This later changed as research findings emerged and my colleagues took the initiative. Since this time we have published over 15 papers and chapters together in UK and European journals and books.

Joint research and publication is a tangible outcome of exchange visits and something that as a psychiatrist from the UK, where we have a culture of research and publication, I was really able to contribute through mentoring and collaborating with colleagues. I also fell in love with the country and built strong friendships which have taken me back to Uganda almost yearly."

Consultant and senior lecturer in social psychiatry

Build up local capacity

Capacity building is a widely used term in development work which can have several different interpretations. Here we take it to mean supporting the development of certain skills or competencies and improving workplace performance. It has two elements: promoting learning through education, and developing talent and leadership to implement changes. The overall aim is to decrease future dependence on external support. By enabling local people to be drivers of change, it promotes the sustainability of overseas work.

You should think about where local people need to gain skills and you can help train them during your placement. It is primarily through these actions that your efforts will endure long after you return home. By supporting the development of skills and competencies coupled with an environment that enables people to put these changes into action, your help will lead to improved workplace performance.

Another important aspect of capacity building and good management is succession planning. Who will do your job after you leave? If you are filling a gap, you will leave a gap after your departure, which will decrease the impact of all your hard work. If you have set up new projects or services, who will run these after you leave?

A long-term placement creates opportunities for you to work closely with local colleagues to ensure that, after your departure, they have the knowledge, skills and capacity to take forward the work that you have started. Don't leave this until the last minute. Trying to hand over a year's worth of work and vision to one person, who already has several responsibilities, in a few hours will not work. Instead, integrate it into your planning from the beginning. Identify people who may be able to take on the work and involve them in the decision-making from the early phases. Be mindful that staff turnover will always happen, so build in a system for those people to train others as well.

"I had a month left of my 6-month placement overseas, and was just beginning to make preparations for my return to the UK. I was working in a district hospital in India but had also started a diabetes service for people in rural areas. I travelled out to them once a week and had built up 15 regular patients: a small number but the service had really changed their lives. If the service stopped it would have a serious and negative impact on their health, but who would continue it after my departure? A committed nurse from the hospital worked with me, but I worried she may not have access to all the resources necessary to continue the service. I had paid our transport out to the rural communities myself (it was only £2 for each journey, which was not a lot to me). The hospital management had also allowed me to take treatment from the hospital out to the communities, but I was not convinced they would allow the nurse to continue doing this in my absence. I realised then that these were all issues we should have discussed right at the start; but my focus then was just on getting the service up and running."

Junior doctor, India

Share your learning

Even if you are not working in research, your learning can make a substantial contribution. Many students publish case reports from their elective experiences. Description of successful techniques or practice can help other clinicians in similar positions, and journals that focus on global health are becoming more common (see Chapter 12). Sharing your findings often has the complementary effect of encouraging and motivating local staff (see case study above). In Chapters 14 and 15 you can find more ideas about how to share your learning with others after your return.

Do not get disheartened

'Change is about evolution not revolution'

It is easy to start with much enthusiasm ('I'm going to turn things around and make the place a success') but then quickly become cynical and disheartened. Change happens slowly. And the pace at which things happen can be different from that in the UK—you might find that some things take a lot longer while other things happen much quicker. How can you manage this slump in enthusiasm?

Assume that making things happen is not going to be easy from the start, and manage your expectations. Prioritise, start small and be focused. Set SMART targets: Specific, Measurable, Achievable, Realistic/Relevant and Time Bound. Change takes time and it is unrealistic to think that it is possible to achieve everything. Go for a few quick wins, to show that change is possible. Small successes may bring about a more positive atmosphere amongst colleagues, and people will gain confidence in the ability to change. Monitoring and evaluating your impact is important, as good results can lift morale and maintain motivation for what is often difficult work.

Big things can make a bigger difference

Although the examples above will all contribute to the impact of your work, a more sustainable change requires a systematic approach. In 2010 the NHS brought out guidelines for effective involvement in international development (Department of Health 2010). The document was aimed primarily at institutional partnerships (Health Links), but the principles they identify are also relevant to all those working to develop and improve services. We explore the most important principles below. Think about how you can incorporate them into your work or organisation.

Guidelines for effective involvement in international development

Any initiative should be:
- Locally owned
- Aligned to local health plans
- Harmonised with other initiatives
- Evidence-based
- Sustainable
- Mutually accountable (responsibility for the project or programme is shared)

The Framework for NHS Involvement in International Development. Department of Health, 2010. *http://www.ihlc.org.uk.*

Locally owned

> "Led and driven by the needs of LMIC, not by the enthusiasm and interests of UK participants. Interventions should be based on written agreements owned by the LMIC partner and avoid 'supply-side driving' (the principle of ownership)."
>
> *Department of Health 2010*

In reality this situation can be rather idealistic. The problem you are trying to address may exist precisely because no one is taking a lead locally. If this is the case, is it right for it to be sidelined?

Any process of change requires an initial catalyst and ownership can happen at many levels. If there is a local champion—someone high up, able to influence others—or someone down the chain but with the drive and time, change may be possible. You may have the opportunity to engage others who share the same vision. All will depend on the length of time you and the local champions have to devote to this and how well it fits with the other principles listed in this section.

So how can you tell if a project you are involved in has or will have local ownership? Ask yourself:

- How was it determined as a priority? Who identified the needs?
- Who are the local champions? What authority do these champions have and what is their commitment to the changes?
- Do incentives exist for individuals to support the change? What reasons exist for people to take responsibility for ensuring the desired change happens?

Alignment

> "Aligned with the government in question's health plans as well as those at district and hospital level (the principle of alignment). This ensures that ownership is encouraged, not by-passed or undermined."
>
> *Department of Health 2010*

Is the change you are trying to bring about in line with national, district and regional health plans? These plans represent the locally identified priorities, a common set of goals to work towards. Monitoring and evaluation may also be easier, as health plans are often tied to a set of measurable indicators, and managers and districts are rewarded if they do well.

You may find that some important issues, which should arguably be priorities, do not feature in the health plans. Health financing constraints simply mean they cannot be prioritised—other conditions may cause higher mortality rates. This is where NGOs and private services sometimes come in: working towards issues that have been neglected by national services.

> "Some doctors are so focused on their own sub-speciality interest or niche area of expertise that they advocate for resources to support it even if it will benefit only a small number of people. It is important to appreciate priorities within the wider health perspective; to be able to do this one needs to step outside one's own narrow speciality or interest."
>
> *Retired neonatologist and project manager*

How do you know if your work is aligned to national policy? Look at government health plans and regional, district or hospital implementation plans. Donors such as DFID also produce country strategies which may be useful. Analyse their budgets as these can be a good indication of where current priorities lie.

> "Our hospital started up a Health Link with the Rural Health Training School in Ghana; the only one of its kind training mid-grade health workers for the whole country. They were training generalists, but career progression was an issue so the government plan was to start offering specialist courses, one of which would be mental health. As we are a mental health trust, we could offer our expertise to develop the new training courses. We read strategic documents and met with a wide range of national, regional and local stakeholders to test the commitment in Ghana to the proposed mental health specialisation. After we had built up a solid relationship with the school and our collaboration had become known to the Ministry of Health, we were asked to assist with curriculum planning. So now the first cohort of students who will become Community Mental Health Workers has started and we are setting the quality through agreed educational standards. While funding is of course an issue, I am sure we will succeed as our work is aligned to national priorities and the mandate of the school."
>
> *Psychiatrist, leading a Health Link with Ghana*

Harmonisation

> "Adequately co-coordinated—with initiatives from other development partners (UK and others) working as one (the principle of harmonisation)."
>
> *Department of Health 2010*

The likelihood is that if you identify something as a problem, others too will have also done so before you. Work together and complement each other's work: you will achieve much more.

Your first impression may be that there is little structure or support within the system, and in some areas you may be starting from scratch. Months later you may be surprised to discover that there is in fact already a committee, organisation, government department or another international donor looking at exactly the same issues that you are trying to address.

How can you ensure your work is harmonised?

- **Spend time fact finding**. What has gone on before you? Don't just limit yourself to your organisation. What are other local facilities and organisations doing in the region? Local colleagues will be privy to much information, so involve them.
- **Map out the key stakeholders** and ask specific questions. For example, what are the donor priorities?
- **Work within existing structures**. If you are based in a large institution, there are also likely to be various committees who may be able to play a role in supporting your work. If you can engage them, you are much more likely to be able to embed your work.

Evidence-based initiatives

"Evidence-based and subject to proper monitoring and evaluation. It is imperative to identify and (wherever possible) measure actual outcomes or results, because so much well-intentioned activity in the past has either done harm or failed to achieve its stated aims."

Department of Health 2010

Ensure that the areas that you are supporting are evidence-based and, if you can, help to promote an interest and access to evidence-based practice and resources. Not only that, but contribute to the evidence base by ensuring monitoring and evaluation is included in your work (see below).

Sources of evidence for interventions

- The Cochrane Library and the Campbell Collaboration produce systematic reviews on the effects of interventions (*http://www.thecochranelibrary.com* and *http://www.campbellcollaboration.org*)
- The HRH Global Resource Center collates publications on human resources for health (health workers) (*http://www.hrhresourcecenter.org/*)
- WHO produces many guidelines and protocols for health work in LMIC (*http://www.who.org*)

"I worked as an orthopaedic surgeon in Malawi for many years. I was also trying to support the development of good orthopaedic services throughout the country and along with other volunteers travelled around to the district hospitals in Malawi providing training to local staff (primarily the orthopaedic clinical officers, OCOs) to cast fractures. The training went well, and all the OCOs had the skills to deal with simple cases, rather than referring them on to the central hospital. However, follow-up visits revealed that a shortage of plaster of Paris and undercast padding at the district hospitals often prevented those who had been trained from doing the work.

I started carrying around large supplies of plaster of Paris and undercast padding with me, distributing it to the district hospitals I visited for follow-up: without them patients with fractures could not be treated. In the short term this helped many patients, but it took me a while to realise that it was a hopeless long-term strategy. I couldn't be the one supplying the whole of Malawi with plaster of Paris! By doing this I was not helping local clinicians develop reliable supply mechanisms.

So I started encouraging local OCOs to lobby their hospital managers, district health officers and the ministry of health to provide a constant supply of plaster of Paris to the district hospitals.

Eventually, after much encouraging, procurement of plaster of Paris became something that district hospitals took responsibility for, rather than relying on visiting surgeons. In this way we were a step closer to bringing about a long-term and sustainable change."

Orthopaedic surgeon, Malawi

Measuring your impact

"If you do not measure results, you cannot tell success from failure,
If you cannot see success, you cannot reward it,
If you cannot reward success, you are probably rewarding failure,
If you cannot see success, you cannot learn from it,
If you cannot recognise failure, you cannot correct it,
If you can demonstrate results, you can win public support."

Adapted by Kusek and Rist (2004) from Osborne and Gaebler (1992)

Monitoring and evaluating your work is integral to its success. The history of development is littered with examples of successes and failures, so learning from your work is important. Monitoring and evaluation (or M&E as it is commonly referred to) is well established in development work, but this format is likely to be unfamiliar to clinical staff. Of course, *monitoring* is inherent in daily clinical work—for example, patients' observations, blood results and supply stores. *Evaluation* is also common, whether clinical audits, staff appraisals or near-miss analyses.

However, M&E is defined slightly differently in development programmes. Successful implementation and outcomes of this type of work can be much less obvious than the cause-and-effect that is the recovery of sick patients. Therefore, you need rigorous M&E to identify and flag up progress and pitfalls, modify work accordingly and show results and failures.

What Is monitoring and evaluation?

Although the term 'monitoring and evaluation' tends to get discussed together as if it is only one thing, M&E are, in fact, two distinct sets of organisational activities, related but not identical.

Monitoring is the systematic collection and analysis of information as a project progresses.

It is aimed at improving the efficiency and effectiveness of a project or organisation. It is based on targets set and activities planned during the planning phases of work. It helps to keep the work on track, and can let management know when things are going wrong. It enables you to determine whether the resources and capacity you have available are sufficient, and whether you are doing what you planned to do.

Evaluation is the comparison of actual project impacts against the agreed strategic plans. It looks at what you set out to do, what you have accomplished and how you accomplished it. It can be formative (taking place during the life of a project) or summative (drawing out learning from a completed project).

Source: Monitoring and Evaluation Toolkit, CIVICUS.

While we will not go into detail here about how to carry out M&E (see box below for further resources), here are some initial questions to think about:

- Who will evaluate the work (internal or external evaluator)?
- What indicators will you look at? Will they be:
  - Qualitative or quantitative?
  - Ones specific to your work, the project as a whole or wider indicators that are already being monitored by the organisation itself? Organisations will often have big goals and will ask you to evaluate the work you do as progress towards achieving them. It is also very helpful to have an evaluation of your work that is meaningful/tangible to you.
- How will you gather the data required (case reports, audits, key informant interviews, focus group discussions and/or cost-effectiveness analyses)?

- How will you disseminate and learn from the evaluation (presentation, writing a paper, stakeholder report)?
- How will this learning be incorporated into future stages of the project?

Project planning and logframes

Most approaches to monitoring and evaluation are based on the project cycle, a framework of learning and action that is widely used by international development agencies, including DFID and the UN agencies. The project cycle is cyclical as the learning from an evaluation feeds into and determines the next stages of a project.

A project planning tool that is widely used is the logical framework analysis (known as a *logframe*) and this is often a donor requirement when applying for funding. This captures the aims, objectives, outcomes and activities of the programme and what indicators will be used to monitor and evaluate them.

Find out more

- *Monitoring and Evaluation (M&E): Some Tools, Methods and Approaches.* World Bank, 2004. *http://www.worldbank.org/ieg*
- *Monitoring and Evaluation Toolkit, CIVICUS. http://www.civicus.org/toolkits/ civicus-planning-toolkits*

Conclusion

This chapter has offered you some key considerations to ensure that your time overseas is of benefit to those you are working with and for. Building capacity through rigorous, sustainable programmes will ensure that your work in international health has maximum impact.

REFERENCES

Awases M, Gbary A, Nyoni J, Chatora R (2004). *Migration of Health Professionals in Six Countries: A Synthesis Report*. Brazzaville: World Health Organization Regional Office for Africa.

Crisp N (2010). *Turning the World Upside Down: The Search for Global Health in the 21st Century*. London: Royal Society of Medicine Press.

Department of Health (2010). *The Framework for NHS Involvement in International Development*. London, Department of Health.

Kusek J, Risk R (2004). *Ten Steps to a Results-Based Monitoring and Evaluation System*. Washington, DC, World Bank.

World Commission on Environment and Development (1987). *Our Common Future*. Oxford, Oxford University Press.

Homecoming

Returning home is not always easy. Indeed, some health workers find this the most difficult aspect of their placement. This final section of the book aims to make your return home as successful as the other parts of your placement.

Chapter 14 (Returning Home) offers personal and professional advice to help you return to UK life. It also gives useful information on how to make your experience relevant for employers and your colleagues in the UK.

Chapter 15 (What Now?) is for those UK health professionals who have completed their placements, but who would like to continue being involved internationally. It describes ways to do this, and gives examples of how other health professionals have achieved this balance.

After reading these chapters, you may feel that returning home need not be the end of your experience. In fact, you might want to use your placement as the beginning of a long and fruitful engagement with global health.

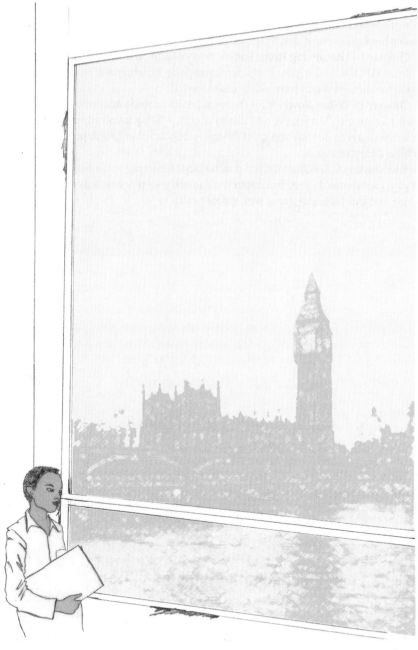

CHAPTER 14

Returning home

You will probably be looking forward to seeing family and friends again, eating familiar food and settling back into UK life. But some aspects of returning home might not be so welcome. Prospective employers or current managers may not appreciate your new-found skills. You may find friends and colleagues less curious about your experiences that you expected. And you may develop psychological or physical symptoms from your time away.

Try to think of this as the final stage of your placement, which will require considerable skill and careful preparation to negotiate successfully. In this chapter, we outline things you can do before and after your return home to make the readjustment easier.

Although there is increasing awareness of the advantages of international health work for the UK, much still needs to be done to ensure that it is properly recognised and valued. Make sure you play your part on your return by publicising your experiences and its benefits to your colleagues, managers and others interested in international work.

Before you leave

In the countdown to your departure date, it is easy to get swept up in a whirlwind of packing, goodbyes and buying presents for those in the UK. Yet these last few weeks can make the difference between a successful return home and a more difficult one. So before you step on that plane, make sure you think about the following:

- **Review your placement.** Have you met your professional and personal objectives? If you made up a personal development plan as discussed in Chapter 12, go over it with your local supervisor. Ask for constructive feedback from your local colleagues (you are more likely to get honest comments face to face). Try to pin down precisely the areas in which you have progressed whilst the experience is still fresh as this will make the framing of these skills back in the UK much easier.

- If you need to **restore your UK registration,** start this process before you leave so that it will be active when you get back to the UK.

- Contact your UK employer or professional association to arrange any **refresher training** that you might need to undertake when you return home.

- As for any job, **tie up any loose ends** before you leave it. Not only is this more professional and lightens the load for the next post-holder, but also it is far easier to do on the ground than trying to finish things off from the UK. People are busy everywhere, and often out of sight can mean out of mind. So make sure you get all forms signed, audits finished and reports submitted before your last day.

- **Identify one or two high-calibre local referees** who know you well and can attest to the roles and responsibilities you have held. Again, it's probably easier to get written references before you leave, than trying to make contact when there's an urgent application deadline coming up.

- If you went with an organisation, **apply for any resettlement grants** available. Getting a job back in the UK can take time and these grants can help cover this limbo period. If you are likely to spend more than a few weeks waiting for a job, try to apply before you get home.

- **Be wary of making promises that are easily broken**. It is likely that you have made many new friends during your time abroad. During the goodbyes, you may make promises to send photos or even help with things like visa applications or reciprocal visits. However, getting back into the whirlwind of UK life may leave you with little time to make good on these promises. Be aware of what you can realistically offer, and try to avoid disappointing those friends who may be waiting hopefully for your reply.

- Finally, gather your thoughts, reflect on your time abroad and **start mentally preparing for the return home.** This is often neglected by returning expatriates and can help prevent reverse culture shock (see below).

Find out more

....

- *End of Assignment Handbook for UN Volunteers*. UNV, September 2009. *http://www.tz.undp.org*. Although designed for UN Volunteers, this Handbook contains useful advice for all expatriates returning home after substantial time abroad. It also considers the process of returning home for those abroad with their partner and/or children.

Readjusting to the UK

Although getting back to your home culture can be a welcome feeling after months as an outsider, it can be more difficult to re-adjust than expected. You might find yourself having to deal with psychological and physical sequelae from your placement. It may take time to feel your usual self and you may have to re-learn ways of working and communicating with people. This section looks at three major types of problem: reverse culture shock, psychological issues and medical problems.

Reverse culture shock

"I have over 20 years' involvement in international health projects in Africa, the Middle East and Asia, but I cannot recall when I last experienced culture shock in any of the countries. However, I always experience reverse culture shock. I find it very difficult coming back, seeing wealth and waste around me and being part of that myself."

Professor of epidemiology and international mental health policy

Many people coming back from mid- to long-term placements experience a degree of *reverse culture shock*. This is similar to normal culture shock, but it is often unanticipated and can cause significant difficulties. Returnees may view UK society with more critical eyes and compare it unfavourably with their host country. Reverse culture shock can also arise from the discrepancy between expatriates' expectations and the reality of life at home. It is easy to idealise the comforts of home and minimise the inconveniences whilst overseas, or expect everything to be the same as when you left. However, you may arrive home to less familiarity than hoped. Family and friends may have their own, new problems, and may not be very interested in your '. . . when I was in Timbuktu' stories. Suddenly, you might find yourself longing to return to your host country, rather than this unfamiliar, unreceptive place.

"I went to Cambodia for 3 months in 2008. I came back and I was full of what I had done, where I had been. But after the initial conversation, most people are not interested any more. Only people that have worked abroad always want to know."

Midwife, Cambodia

Reverse culture shock has the same stages as normal culture shock: initial euphoria, then irritability, hostility and low moods, and finally re-adjustment and re-engagement. Generally, the more adapted to your life overseas, the more difficult your re-insertion will be. Other factors that can affect the degree of reverse culture shock include: the degree of cultural difference between your home culture and the host culture, how long you were away, previous overseas experience, and your reasons for returning (UNV 2009).

Anticipation and preparation can be effective in preventing or mitigating reverse culture shock. Before you leave, ask yourself whether your expectations of home are realistic—try to remember some of the daily stresses you faced before. Approach your move home as you would another placement. Read up on changes that have occurred since you've been gone (for example, politically or in your local area). Finally, plan ways to relate your experiences to people other than just your immediate friends—for example, your funders or an international interest group.

> "After 2 months in Zambia, when I arrived home, I was very emotional for a couple of weeks. I felt I wanted to share my experience with people, so worked on putting together a presentation and sorting my pictures for the people that have helped fund my placement and helped me with planning. Doing something concrete made me feel a lot better."
>
> *Ophthalmic nurse, Zambia*

Psychological issues

An intense experience abroad combined with reverse culture shock can easily lead to psychological distress. This may be more relevant to those who have been working in humanitarian emergencies, where they may have come into direct contact with traumatic situations—violence, hunger, fear, disease or death—and not yet come to terms with what they witnessed. Other experiences—such as a high workload, team conflict, relationship problems, guilt or a loss of ideals—can make it difficult to cope. It is not unusual to return home and find yourself overwhelmed by recent experiences.

If you are finding things difficult, do share your feelings with your family and friends. Although they may not be able to empathise with your experiences, talking it through can help to feel less isolated.

It is also useful to stay in touch with people who have had similar experiences. Some organisations may even be able to organise psychological assessment and/or counselling for returned volunteers and it is something you can bring up during a debriefing session. Having the opportunity to talk and share your experiences with someone—whether a professional therapist or peer—can help you start the recovery process.

> "I went to Cambodia for 3 months in 2008. My placement was arranged by NHS Education South Central. After my return, as part of the programme's protocol, I was asked to do psychological testing twice: immediately after returning and again after 6 months. It was comforting to know that the means to address psychological problems were available if I needed them."
>
> *Midwife, Cambodia*

> "My parents are quite supportive of my work, but they are not crazy about it. I keep a little distance between home (family and friends) and work. My family and friends do not understand many of the things that I want to talk about, and also there are many things that you can't tell them. I've made peace in my mind and I have accepted this fact."
>
> *Nurse, MSF*

Do seek professional help if you are suffering from:

- **Persistent low mood**. Up to 60% of aid workers describe predominantly negative emotions on their return home, and over 30% report depression (CDC, 2010). Contributory factors include the 'loss' of your life and status overseas and a sense of isolation from friends and peers, often combined with a period of unemployment and uncertainty. If your low mood is persistent, do visit your GP.
- **Symptoms of post-traumatic stress disorder**. These can include nightmares, flashbacks, emotional numbness and finding it hard to relax or sleep. If you witnessed or were involved in any distressing incidents or were under continuous stress, you are at increased risk of post-traumatic stress disorder. Seek help through your organisation or GP in the first place.

Medical problems

Diseases picked up during your time overseas can present after you return home. Of note, *Plasmodium falciparum* malaria can present up to 1 year after infection, and longer intervals have been recorded for the relapsing strains. If you've been in an endemic zone, be alert to any fever or flu-like symptoms and flag up your time overseas if you require investigation. Many returnees opt for screening for tropical disease on their return home. This is offered by many travel clinics as a service (see the International Society of Travel Medicine's website for an online directory of UK travel clinics: http://www.istm.org).

Physical and emotional tiredness are normal after a tough placement, so try to put aside a couple of weeks when you return before starting work. Remember that tiredness and apathy can be symptoms of tropical infections, reverse culture shock and/or depression, so do see your GP if it lasts longer that you would expect.

Getting your career back on track

> "We will work closely with the Department of Health to ensure that where possible any health professionals who practice temporarily in the developing world will not be disadvantaged in terms of their career progression."
>
> *One World Conservatism: A Conservative Agenda for International Development, October 2009*

It's hard not to feel that your career has been derailed slightly when coming back to the UK after time abroad. Your peers have progressed up the ladder, you're feeling rusty in UK practice, and no-one seems to appreciate that you learnt quite a bit overseas. Whether you're looking for a new job or returning to an old post, framing your newly acquired skills and experiences will be key to proving that your time overseas had value and requires recognition.

> "Very soon after my return from Tanzania I was called for a job interview. I didn't get the job and it was quite upsetting. They did not ask me about my experience in Africa, although the job involved working with refugees. I realised that in Tanzania I had been constantly simplifying things. The result was that in this interview I may not have expressed myself in the sophisticated manner they were expecting. It was very disappointing."
>
> *Psychologist, Tanzania*

Making the most of your new skills and experience

> "Through this work, we can play our part in improving health globally while developing leadership and other skills in the NHS and further building and sustaining our international networks."
>
> *Sir David Nicholson, NHS Chief Executive (England), Framework for NHS Involvement in International Development, Department of Health 2010*

Ensuring that your time overseas is valued and recognised is an integral part of your placement. To do so, you will need to frame or 'sell' your skills and experience in a way that is relevant to your current or potential employer and your regulatory body.

Understand how your experience relates to current UK policy on international development and health. This will enable you to answer questions about your reasons for working overseas and how it benefits the UK. Be familiar with policy such as the Department of Health's *Framework for NHS Involvement in International Development* (2010) and the NHS Staff Council's *Agenda for Change* (2011). Both documents affirm the benefit of work overseas for the UK health sector, and include guidance for employers on acknowledging your international role. Appendix 1 lists further key documents.

Then match the new skills you have gained overseas to a skills and competency framework. Use the framework that is most suited to your profession and stage of career—ask your manager or peers for advice. For each competency listed, describe concrete examples of how you demonstrated this whilst you were overseas. Back these up with evidence from your portfolio (see Chapter 12). Try the framework shown in Figure 14.1 as a template.

If you are returning to a post, share your matched framework and portfolio with your line manager and more senior professionals if possible. This will help you to gain recognition for your placement overseas and may smooth the way for others keen

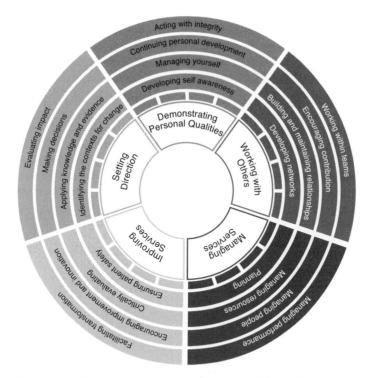

Outer ring labels (clockwise from top):
Acting with integrity
Continuing personal development
Managing yourself
Developing self awareness
Building and maintaining relationships
Encouraging contribution
Working within teams
Developing networks
Managing performance
Managing people
Managing resources
Planning
Facilitating transformation
Encouraging improvement and innovation
Critically evaluating
Ensuring patient safety
Identifying the contexts for change
Applying knowledge and evidence
Making decisions
Evaluating impact

Inner segments:
Demonstrating Personal Qualities
Setting Direction
Working with Others
Managing Services
Improving Services

Figure 14.1 Baseline core competencies for all health professionals with over 2 years' relevant post-graduate experience. © NHS Institute for Innovation and Improvement and Academy of Medical Royal Colleges 2010.

to engage in international work. If you are applying for jobs, tailor your CV to these competencies and use your examples in application forms if possible. Bring your framework and portfolio to interviews.

> "Ultimately people going abroad should be proud of what they are doing and face interview panels with confidence. People respect that."
>
> *Junior doctor, Egypt*

It can be hard to convey to your peers, managers and potential employers just how your experience abroad relates to your work in the UK. Try to be business-like about it. Always mention your competencies, what you learnt and your responsibilities during your placement. Use examples that they can relate to easily. For example, 'It was like working for this hospital, with a similar catchment area and target population, but with only 200 trained health professionals'. Finally, be subtly proactive. Seek out opportunities to tell your line manager and colleagues how your experience overseas has helped you in your current role.

Refresher training

> "When an NHS employee returns to work after an employment break of 12 months or longer their manager, in agreement with the employee, may put in place training arrangements for re-introduction to the workplace. For career breaks of less than 12 months, an appropriate re-orientation or induction may be proposed and should be agreed by close consultation between employer and employee."
>
> BMA, *Broadening Your Horizons*, 2009

If you are returning to your old position after a medium- or long-term placement, then you will probably have to undergo some refresher training. This could be anything from a re-orientation session to a longer programme for retraining in certain skills. Ensure that this training only covers areas of UK practice in which you may have become rusty. If you have been using certain skills to a high standard overseas, then there is no need for you to be re-trained in these areas. There may also be learning programmes run by your professional association or Royal College that might help your return to practice.

Sharing your experiences

There are an increasing number of ways in which you can share your experiences with others. In fact, the dissemination of learning and new skills is one of the ways that international work can be justified for UK health professionals—so try to make it a priority.

- If your professional association has an **international office**, get in touch with them (see Appendix 1). They might keep a database of people like you who can contribute to projects and respond to international requests for help.

> "I try to get my experience valued in the UK by keeping in touch with the agencies I work with such as the Royal College of Nursing and the THET. This has worked because, among other things, they have invited me to speak at their events about my work overseas. I also have been asked for my advice and input to help some of these organisations develop nurse leadership programmes."
>
> *Nurse manager and consultant, Tanzania/Somaliland*

- Give **presentations** on where you've been and what you've done to relevant groups. People who may be interested include: your colleagues, your Trust board, any international groups you belong to, and anyone who has funded you. Not only will this improve your presentation skills, but it will also raise the profile of international work.

- Write **articles** on your experiences or your programme for health journals and magazines, or even local newspapers. This is an excellent way of recording the significance and impact of your work overseas. Professional associations and colleges such as the BMA, RCN and RCM encourage health professionals to share their experience through their publications and web forums.

- Submit a presentation for your professional association/college's **annual conference**. For example, the RCM annual conference or student midwives conference.

- Contribute to **online forums** set up by international volunteer organisations and networks. These will enable you to support others working in the same country or the same field. In most cases, you do not need to work for an organisation to join its forums.

- Finally, **share your experiences with your hosts**. Send them a copy of any reports you write and any photographs you took during your placement. These are usually much appreciated and can facilitate further placements from UK health professionals.

Find out more

....

Some online forums

- VSO community: *http://www.community.vsointernational.org/*
- International Forum on Development Service: *http://forum-ids.org/*
- IDEAS Forum (Scotland): *http://www.ideas-forum.org.uk/*
- Doctors.net.uk: *http://www.doctors.net.uk/*
- Aid worker exchanges: *http://www.aidworkers.net/*

Conclusion

Returning to the UK is the final part of your placement. It might not be straightforward and re-immersion into your personal and professional life back home can be difficult. If you can overcome this, then the next and final chapter gives you ideas on how to continue to be involved in international work.

REFERENCES

British Medical Association International Department (2009). *Broadening Your Horizons: A Guide to Taking Time Out to Work and Train in Developing Countries.* London: BMA.

Centers for Disease Control and Prevention (2010). *The Yellow Book: Health Information for International Travel.* Atlanta: CDC.

Department of Health (2010). *The Framework for NHS Involvement in International Development.* London: Department of Health.

NHS Institute for Innovation and Improvement and the Academy of Medical Colleges. *Medical Leadership Competency Framework.* http://www.institute. nhs.uk/assessment_tool/general/medical_leadership_competency_ framework_-_homepage.html

NHS Staff Council (2011). *Agenda for Change: NHS Terms and Conditions for Service Handbook.* Amendment Number 23. Pay Circular (AforC) 2/2011.

One World Conservatism: A Conservative Agenda for International Development. Policy Green Paper No. 11. October 2009. http://www.conservatives.com

United Nations Volunteers (2009). *End of Assignment Handbook for UN Volunteers.* Geneva: United Nations.

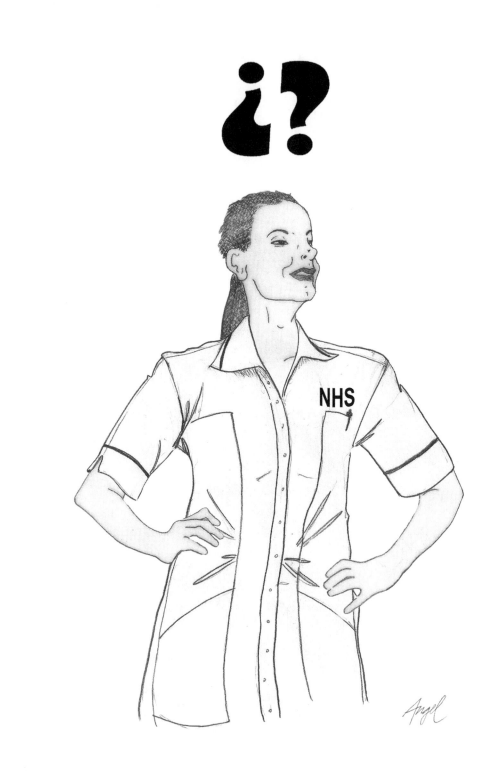

CHAPTER 15

What now?

Most UK health professionals who go overseas find the experience life-changing. Although they may return to their careers in the UK, they often want to retain links to their projects abroad or stay involved in global health issues.

This last chapter offers ideas on how to do this. The first part outlines possible ways to combine international work with a UK career. The second part looks at how you can retain an international focus but without the travel. The final section shares some stories from those 'bitten by the bug' who decided to make it their full-time career.

Combining work in the UK and overseas

Become part of a health link

Health Links (described in Chapter 4) are very inclusive, with participants including clinicians, managers, academics and support staff. If your expertise is relevant to the work of a Health Link, you might be involved in one-off or regular targeted short-term visits (2- to 3-week) to the overseas partner institution as well as hosting staff from the partner institution back in the UK.

There are over 100 institutional health partnerships between UK organisations and their southern counterparts. If your institution is already involved in one, you might be able to contribute relevant expertise. But if not, you could think about starting one. Many Health Links are in fact initiated by people who were previously engaged in international work. THET and the IHLC offer information on existing Links and how to start one up, including information on how to find a suitable partner institution.

Find out more

....

- Tropical Health and Education Trust: *http://www.thet.org*
- International Health Links Centre: *http:// www.ihlc.org.uk*

Michael Roe works as a consultant paediatrician in an NHS Trust. He has assisted with establishing and developing a health partnership between his own NHS Trust, a sister organisation in northern Ghana and a UK-based NGO.

"As a medical student, I experienced development work in Thailand. Once I qualified as a doctor, I wanted to undertake humanitarian assistance. I passed my MRCP and then worked for an NGO for two-and-a-half years, including trips to Afghanistan and the Democratic Republic of Congo. After this time, I wanted to settle down and refocus on my UK-based career and become a consultant. Having achieved that, I looked for opportunities to use my past experiences and expertise, acknowledging my passion and interest in health in LMIC. I was introduced to the idea of setting up a partnership with health organisations in Ghana and this appeared to be the right project for me to be involved with. There was a need for a paediatric lead and preferably someone with previous experience. The partnership has developed a framework for its activities and plans to be a long-term project. The Trust supports this work and has facilitated me and other colleagues to begin to achieve our set objectives."

Volunteer with an international organisation

"I am trying to do international health work without having to be overseas for long periods of time. I have a family in the UK and also I have a responsibility to my patients here. However, I find that most volunteer organisations are not interested in people like me and tend to offer support only to those who can go overseas for long periods of time. It is really frustrating because I have international experience, with the Red Cross and other well-known organisations. I have experience and skills to contribute."

Anaesthetist, Afghanistan/Nepal/Ghana

Whilst there are many more opportunities for medium- and long-term placements, organisations will still be looking for those with particular skills for short-term placements. Such organisations include Operation Smile, Mercy Ships, Orbis and several other smaller-scale 'fly-in-and-operate' initiatives. If you have the right skills (usually surgical and anaesthetic) you will be very valuable to them and will often be asked to go on repeat missions. Chapter 7 has more information on these organisations.

Maintain your overseas contacts

The relationships that are most appreciated by overseas colleagues are those that have longevity. So while your 2-year stint may have ended, there might still be a role for to fulfil once a year, a couple of weeks at a time. And it will be much easier for you to do this as you know the context and have built up trusts and friendship.

This type of work is arranged directly with your overseas organisation and could involve coming in to teach specific modules, examining, delivering training, providing support in workshops, following up on research or delivering specific services that are not locally available (e.g. hernia surgery). If you know you want to continue to stay engaged, explore these possibilities with colleagues and management before you leave, and you might maintain a lifelong engagement with them.

Develop an international dimension to your job

Introducing an international dimension into your job is not an easy task, but it is possible. First, enquire about existing opportunities at your workplace. Assess if you could add value to any existing initiatives, and build up your case for working with them. Alternatively, if you can show how your present role could address both national and global priorities, you might find a way to incorporate this into your current post.

Dr Gwyneth Lewis OBE was the clinical director for international maternal health at the Department of Health, London. Gwyneth is especially well known for editing and implementing the WHO manual *Beyond the Numbers* which promotes mortality and morbidity reviews of maternal deaths in over 58 countries around the world.

"I first got involved in international work, and the work of WHO in particular, in the 1980s when I ran the HIV/AIDS unit for DH. It was then that I became increasingly aware of the burden of international health and the invisibility, at that time, of women and children's health issues.

As part of my professional development, DH enabled me to undertake additional training in public health. It was then that my real passion for working towards increasing the profile and the need to urgently reduce the over 7 million avoidable deaths which occur to mothers and newborns around the world as a result of pregnancy-related complications. This is the largest inequalities gap in

➲

the world. I raised the issues whenever and wherever I could. I joined organisations to provide help but it wasn't enough. I was lucky to arrange a secondment to the Making Pregnancy Safer programme at the WHO and worked with them part time for some years. DH enabled me to do this because they recognised that the work we do in the UK to improve maternal health can contribute to the work that is needed in other countries. Many countries have requested help in setting up safer maternity services and audits, and it has been an honour to help them.

I couldn't have done all of this without support from my employers, who understood how our work in the UK can contribute to the UK's global health strategy. I knew I was representing the NHS and the Department of Health when I worked abroad, and it made me very proud. We have a lot to share."

If you are undertaking significant international work in your job, lobby your line manager to get it written into your job description. This will allow you to justify the time spent and may make the juggling act easier.

Finally, if the above measures fail or you still feel unfulfilled with the balance of national to international work in your life, consider applying for posts that have a specific international component.

Before joining the Royal College of Midwives, **Sue Jacob** had been a midwife and midwife teacher in Manchester and London. Her role at the RCM focuses on developing guidance tools for prospective and current midwifery students and those returning to practice, and supporting the development and recognition of midwifery education around the world.

"We work to influence policy in countries around the world. One of my first overseas engagements was in Indonesia. We had been asked to help in their needs assessments of midwifery education in the country. Our work with our Indonesian sister organisations resulted in the introduction of clinical training in decision-making, particularly targeted to those working in the most hard to reach areas."

Start up your own organisation

Many people return from visits overseas with an understanding of where gaps exist and a vision of what they could do to fill these gaps. This might involve mobilising financial support or expertise from the UK to make a difference overseas.

If you feel strongly that you have found an issue that no-one is addressing or a viable solution to a problem your colleagues overseas are facing, and you have the skills, contacts, time and motivation to continue offering support, starting up your own organisation might be the right option. Before you start, make sure that no-one is already doing what you plan to—if so, it is much better to work with them than to duplicate work.

"During a trip to Malawi, I visited the national medical school. I found that many of the talented students from poorer families were struggling and even having to drop out of medical school due to lack of funding. So I set up Medic to Medic, a scheme which helps health workers through their training by guaranteeing tuition fees and other costs. UK doctors donate financially and are also linked to individual students, whom they mentor through medical school. The idea is simple, but it has helped many students through their studies both in Malawi and now Uganda."

Dr Kate Mandeville, http://www.medictomedic.org.uk

To set up a charity, visit the website of the Charity Commission at http://www.charity-commission.gov.uk. This offers useful advice on what to consider before starting up a charity and an overview of the whole process. To set up your own company, start by visiting Business Link (http://www.businesslink.gov.uk).

Staying in the UK

Now that you've returned from your overseas stint, you may need to stay in the UK for the foreseeable future for personal or professional reasons. How can you put your hard-earned international experience to good use without leaving the country?

Inspire others to get involved in international work

The difficulty for many young health workers coming through the system is that they cannot envisage how to combine their UK career with international work. They need more visible role models and prominent professionals to speak up for the merits of working overseas and to demonstrate that going overseas will not be the end of your career in the UK. You could be this ambassador for international work. For example, you could:

- Offer to **speak about your experiences** at your local training institution or a careers fair. Professional bodies such as the Royal Colleges and other organisations frequently run conferences with a global health focus.
- **Write articles** about your work overseas and how it was possible for you. Target student or university publications.
- **Contact Alma-Mata**. This is an organisation working to increase post-graduate training in global health. They run conferences and career days and are looking for speakers.

Raise awareness of global health issues

Through your experiences, you will have observed first-hand the conditions facing many individuals in poor countries. This knowledge can be used to promote change though advocacy efforts. Use your influence to speak up for those whose voice is not always heard, especially in the UK.

Just by talking to your friends about your experience overseas, you have already engaged in some simple advocacy. You can increase the impact of your advocacy by either talking to more people or by talking to more powerful people. Many NGOs run advocacy campaigns which you can support, or you can try out some of our suggestions below:

- When the **media** publish articles that misrepresent situations or over-simplify things, write to them. Your answer might be published and help increase understanding.
- Participate in **forums** such as HIFA-2015, with over 3,000 registered members from 150 countries sharing information about their experiences in LMIC—from the benefits of community health workers to the use of traditional medicines. This forum is also used by the WHO and other organisations for consultations. There is also a sister forum, CHILD-2015, focused on child health. http:www.hifa2015.org.
- You may have found during the placement that certain **clinical guidelines** have become obsolete. If so, write to the person or organisation that promotes the guidelines and suggest your changes.
- **Write a guide or book** about a topic you think needs to be addressed. *Turning the World Upside Down: The Search for Global Health in the 21st Century* by Nigel Crisp (2010) is an example.

"When I was in Central Asia I can remember the number of occasions in which I needed professional supervision or to ask a clinical question to someone that could give me an answer. I remember a boy having epileptic fits and we did not have the medicines to treat him. It would have helped us to have access to senior and experienced health professionals, particularly specialists in the UK. For this reason, upon my return I tried to encourage my organisation to set up a UK support network for health professionals during their placement."

Paediatrician, Afghanistan

Mentor, teach and provide support

There is ample opportunity and need to support others in the sector: either fellow UK professionals working in the field or former local colleagues. With technology advances and increasing access to the internet, you could set up regular sessions with a colleague overseas to discuss cases or offer support. See box below for an innovative example.

"Every Friday, 30 newly qualified doctors in Somaliland sit in front of their computers and are taught by some of the best clinical minds in London—one week a surgeon, one week a mental health specialist, another a physician.

The young African medics have already uploaded their clinical cases, so the teachers offer interactive, 'hands-on' practical tuition over the worldwide web. Earlier in the week, the same doctors have spent time on the internet with King's [College] medical students, passing on expert knowledge from their homeland. This is global health in action."

Extract from Thornton (2010) Global health—it's not just malaria,
The Guardian, 14 June 2010
See also the work of the NGO MedicineAfrica (http://www.medicineafrica.com)

If you went through or are affiliated to a UK organisation, you could mentor new recruits and pass on the knowledge gained through your experience. If your organisation doesn't arrange UK mentorship yet, suggest it as a useful resource.

Staying engaged with your organisation

Some volunteer organisations have been more successful than others at developing useful ways to engage their recruits post-placement. VSO, for example, has developed a forum, VSO Community, where current and former volunteers can share experiences and learning (*http://community.vsointernational.org/*). Other organisations keep a bureau of speakers willing to share their experiences at recruitment days, training or PR events. Find out what your organisation does and how you can stay involved with them.

There are also an increasing number of university global health courses, and your expertise may be of value to them. Explore the possibility of giving a one-off talk or seminar, or even teaching a specific module or series of lectures.

Skillshare is also committed to building understanding of international development issues in the UK, and has worked with different medical schools including Leicester, Nottingham, Swansea and the Faculty of Medicine at Trinity College Dublin, designing and teaching special study modules on Global Health and Development. Returned development workers and health trainers have the opportunity to deliver a session to medical students based on their experience overseas, helping students to prepare and understand the global determinants of health and development.

Support a link or partnership

Even without going on visits, there is plenty of work to be done for Health Links, Community Links and School Links. Work such as coordination, needs assessment, advocacy, fundraising and planning visits is better done by people who understand the context and the challenges of working overseas.

In addition to Health Links, there are about 300 communities in Britain linked with other communities around the world, including school twinning projects. Some of these community and school partnerships are involved in health work, others in many other worthwhile causes such as promoting awareness of fair trade products and encouraging donations for disasters. Find out more about how you could get involved at UK One World Linking Association (*http://www.ukowla.org.uk*), which is the umbrella organisation for all school and community links.

PONT is a community to community link between Rhondda Cynon Taf in South Wales and a district in Uganda called Mbale that was set up in 2005. Within the link there are 13 different categories of partnerships such as engineering, churches, police, environment, schools and health.

The health aspect of the link involves both primary and secondary care. Health professionals from the hospitals in both Wales and Uganda are involved. They work in collaboration with local NGOs in Uganda to deliver training to 450 community health workers and the distribution of mosquito nets in Mbale.

This link was awarded two UN Gold Star awards for excellence in community linking, in recognition of its work. It is one of only two projects in the world to receive such an award.

Full-time work in international health

After the excitement, challenges, lifestyle and opportunities of working overseas, the idea of returning full time to the UK may seem unappealing. Why not work in international health full time? You will have to weigh up the pros and cons carefully; however, there are many opportunities available if you decide this is the right move. Chapter 7 lists organisations that are likely to have full-time openings available.

Work for international organisations

If you want to do this full time, you can either take on consecutive short-term assignments or move over into the organisation's administration team on a permanent contract. The former can mean a lot of job applications and little job security, but a very diverse lifestyle. Once you build up experience in the field, you are likely to fit the profile of exactly who these organisations are looking to recruit, so it usually won't be too hard to find a job.

"I first started working overseas in 1974. I took this step partly because I didn't feel I would be an academic doctor nor that I fitted into the UK system too well. My first job overseas was as head of department in the Fiji medical school (I was the only member of the department) and I had a wonderful 3 years teaching small classes of students and doing interesting surgery. I then worked with the UK ODA (now DFID) who sent me to the idyllic locations of Vanuatu, Seychelles, Kenya. But ODA then started moving into public health and population planning rather than providing medical specialists, so in 1982 I decided to broaden my horizon and that is when I took up my first job with the Red Cross. I have now been on over 30 overseas missions with them.

I have also worked with MSF and done some training and locum work back in the UK. It has been a lot of job applications, and working on contract means that one has no job security. But in 35 years, apart from a few stray months which I accepted as holiday, I have never been unemployed."

Surgeon

Many organisations also recruit health professionals onto the management and advisory teams to oversee projects. This may mean a move away from direct clinical work towards management, but can result in an interesting career overseas.

Work for local organisations

If you want to work full time in international health for a local organisation, there are numerous opportunities. As we have discussed, many hospitals and health training institutions are desperate to recruit people with the right competencies to fill their vacancies. This can be on a local salary, but some governments and organisations may top this up if you are an international candidate.

You could also think about starting up your own practice or organisation in an LMIC.

In 1959 Reginald and Catherine Hamlin, two gynaecologists, arrived in Addis Ababa to open a midwifery school. They planned to stay for 3 years. On the evening of their arrival a fellow gynaecologist came to visit and described obstetric fistulae to the Hamlins, neither of whom had ever seen one before. 'To us they were an academic rarity', Catherine recalls. A fistula is caused by unrelieved obstructed labour and causes incontinence, leading young women to be shunned by their family. At the time there was no treatment for obstetric fistula anywhere in the world. The Hamlins went on to pioneer fistula repair surgery and in 1974 opened the Addis Ababa Fistula Hospital. It remains the only medical centre in the world dedicated

➲

exclusively to fistula repair. Catherine Hamlin has numerous humanitarian awards and has been nominated for the Nobel Peace Prize.

Adapted from Hamlin (2004) The Hospital by the River: A Story of Hope. http://www.fistulafoundation.org

Become a consultant

Once you have built up experience of working overseas, you may have a role to play as a consultant, advising and designing particular aspects of health care interventions.

Liz Ollier undertook VSO before becoming an NHS national trainee. Early in her career she spent some time working in Iran, but returned to pursue her career as a manager, culminating in a Chief Executive post. In her late 40s she wanted a career change and resigned, to work independently both in the UK and overseas. She has worked both through a specialist health development consultancy company (HLSP) and directly for organisations including WHO, bilateral donors and NGOs. As well as evaluating and implementing health interventions in low income countries across the world, Liz is a non-executive Director of the Norfolk and Norwich University Hospitals NHS Foundation Trust.

"I mostly work at strategic level on health systems in LMIC. It is easy to underestimate the learning that you need to do to get involved in global health work. The work that I do now is in a different context and requires a different knowledge set. I had to learn about the aid environment, about different governance structures and funding mechanisms, about the impact of tropical and infectious diseases. So I felt that there was relatively little I could bring from my NHS experience apart from my management skills. Financially, I might have been better off in the NHS; just marginally but there have been other rewards.

I think my international experience brings something back to the NHS. I have now a greater understanding of health economics, monitoring and evaluation. My assumptions about health workforce issues have been challenged for the better. I also have a greater knowledge of research, both clinically but also in relation to health systems. The work I do is challenging, but always different and rewarding."

A final conclusion

Working internationally will be an experience that will be with you forever. You might do it as a one-off experience or plan to stay involved, in different guises and degrees, for the rest of your life. In this book we hope you have found the information to make this experience successful for you, for your hosts and for the wider picture. The visibility of health professionals with successful international experience is slowly increasing and international work is finally becoming more accepted in the NHS. Continue this change by being an ambassador for international work.

> "Although sometimes I can be the most cynical about this [international health] work, I know it is one of the best things I have done in my life. I have not changed the world but I have changed myself in ways I would have never imagined. I believe for the better."
>
> *Paediatrician, Afghanistan/the Democratic Republic of Congo/Ghana*

REFERENCES

Crisp N (2010). *Turning the World Upside Down: The Search for Global Health in the 21st Century*. London: Royal Society of Medicine Press.

Hamlin C (2004). *The Hospital by the River: A Story of Hope*. Toronto: Monarch Books.

Thornton J (2010). Global health—it's not just malaria. *The Guardian*, 14 June 2010. http://www.guardian.co.uk/journalismcompetition/global-health-its-not-just-malaria.

Appendix 1

Useful contacts

Royal Colleges and international departments

Many of the Royal Colleges have international departments which coordinate the colleges' international work overseas and provide policy and guidance. Some also have their own projects.

The International Forum of the Academy of Medical Royal Colleges (AoMRC)
Asterisks below denote members of the International Forum of AoMRC
The Forum aims to bring together those involved in international activity from medical, nursing, industrial and NGOs. It aims to coordinate the international activities of the Royal Colleges.

http://www.rcif.org.uk

Royal College of Surgeons of England*
Including the Faculty of Dental Surgery
http://www.rcseng.ac.uk/international

Royal College of Surgeons of Edinburgh*
http://www.rcsed.ac.uk

Association of Surgeons of Great Britain and Ireland
http://www.asgbi.org.uk

Royal College of Radiologists*
http://www.rcr.ac.uk

Royal College of Psychiatrists*
http://www.rcpsych.ac.uk

Royal College of Physicians and Surgeons of Glasgow*
http://www.rcpsglasg.co.uk

Royal College of Physicians of Ireland*
http://www.rcpi.ie

Royal College of Paediatrics and Child Health*
http://www.rcpch.ac.uk

Royal College of Pathologists*
http://www.rcpath.org

Royal College of Ophthalmologists*
http://www.rcophth.ac.uk

Royal College of Physicians*
International Department
http://www.rcplondon.ac.uk/international/

Faculty of Public Health*
Faculty of the Royal College of Physicians
http://www.fph.org.uk/international

Royal College of Obstetricians and Gynaecologists*
http://www.rcog.org.uk/international

Royal College of Anaesthetists*
http://www.rcoa.ac.uk

Royal College of General Practitioners*
http://www.rcgp.org.uk/international

Royal College of Nursing*
International Department
http://www.rcn.org.uk/

Royal College of Midwives*
International Office
http://www.rcm.org.uk

Royal Pharmaceutical Society of Great Britain
http://www.rpsgb.org.uk

Royal College of Speech and Language Therapists
http://www.rcslt.org

Professional associations with an international focus

British Medical Association
International Department
http://www.bma.org.uk/international

ADAPT
Specialist interest group for chartered physiotherapists in international health and development
http://www.adapt-physio.org.uk

International Working Group of the British Association of Occupational Therapists
http://www.baot.org.uk

Imaging in Developing Countries Special Interest Group of the Society and College of Radiographers
A network of radiographers and other professionals who are working together to support the advancement of radiography in developing countries
http://www.idcsig.org

Communication Therapy International
Set up by a group of UK speech and language therapists for those interested in working in communication disabilities overseas
http://www.commtherapyint.com

International Orthoptic Association (IOA) representative of the British and Irish Orthoptic Society
The IOA links international requests for orthoptists with volunteers in member countries. Information on the IOA volunteer programme can be obtained from the IOA representative at the British and Irish Orthoptic Society
http://www.orthoptics.org.uk

ALMA MATA Global Health Network
Network for doctors in training and medical students who are passionate about international health
http://www.almamata.net

MedSIN
Network of medical students with an interest in international health, with branches at universities across the UK
http://www.medsin.org

Department of Health—Global Health Team
http://www.dh.gov.uk/en/healthcare/international/globalhealth/index.htm

Regulatory bodies

General Medical Council
http://www.gmc-uk.org

Nursing and Midwifery Council
http://www.nmc-uk.org

General Pharmaceutical Council
http://www.pharmacyregulation.org

General Dental Council
http://www.gdc-uk.org

Health Professions Council
http://www.hpc-uk.org

Practicalities

NHS Pensions
http://www.nhsbsa.nhs.uk/pensions

NHS Employers
http://www.nhsemployers.org

NHS Jobs
NHS Jobs is the dedicated online recruitment service for the NHS
http://www.jobs.nhs.uk

Her Majesty's Revenue & Customs Residency Department
Handles tax enquiries for most people not resident in the UK who receive income from
a source in the UK or pay UK National Insurance Contributions
http://www.hmrc.gov.uk/cnr

Foreign and Commonwealth Office
List details of all foreign Embassies and High Commissions in the UK, UK diplomatic
posts abroad, the LOCATE service, passport enquiries and travel advice by country
http://www.fco.gov.uk

Council of International Schools
Accredits international schools worldwide and contains a directory of international
schools in more than 100 countries
http://www.cois.org/

Travel health

International Society of Travel Medicine
Provides an online directory of global travel clinics
http://www.istm.org

National Travel Health Network and Centre (NaTHNaC)
Provides country-specific information, disease outbreak reports and general health advice
http://www.nathnac.org

InterHealth
Provides a one-stop travel clinic service by appointment
http://www.interhealth.org.uk/

TravelPharm
An independent pharmacy based in Derbyshire which provides competitively priced antimalarials and other travel products such as mosquito nets, sun block and water purification tablets
http://www.travelpharm.com

UK linking organisations

International Health Links Centre
http://www.ihlc.org.uk

Tropical Health and Education Trust
http://www.thet.org

UK One World Linking Association
http://www.ukowla.org.uk

Welsh for Africa Health Links Network
http://www.wales.nhs.uk/sites3/home.cfm?orgid=834

Network of International Development Organisations in Scotland
http://www.nidos.org.uk

Research organisations and funders

The Wellcome Trust
http://www.wellcome.ac.uk

Medical Research Council
http://www.mrc.ac.uk

The Nuffield Foundation
http://www.nuffieldfoundation.org

London School of Hygiene and Tropical Medicine
http://www.lshtm.ac.uk

Liverpool School of Tropical Medicine
http://www.liv.ac.uk

Nuffield Centre for International Health and Development
http://www.leeds.ac.uk/nuffield

UCL Institute for Global Health
http://www.ucl.ac.uk/global-health

Appendix 2

Useful resources

Generic information

Key UK publications

- Crisp N (2007). *Global Health Partnerships: The UK Contribution to Health in LMIC (The Crisp Report)*. http://www.dh.gov.uk/.
- Department of Health (2008). *Global Health Partnerships: The UK Contribution to Health in LMIC—The Government Response*. Product no.286615. http://www.dh.gov.uk.
- Department of Health (2008). *Health Is Global: A UK Government Strategy 2008–13*. http://www.dh.gov.uk.
- DFID (2009). *Eliminating World Poverty: Building our Common Future (White Paper)*. http://www.dfid.gov.uk/documents.
- NHS and Department of Health (2010). *The Framework for NHS Involvement in International Development*. http://www.ihlc.org.uk.

UK support for international work

- Banatvala N, Macklow-Smith A (1997). Bringing it back to Blighty. *British Medical Journal* 314:S2-7094.
- Banatvala N, Scott I (2001). Working overseas: from individual to organisational strategy. *British Medical Journal* 323:2.
- BMA International Department (2007). *Improving Health for the World's Poor: What Can Health Professionals Do?* http://www.bma.org.uk/international/globalhealth/.

Global health

- *Council on International Relations Global Governance Monitor.* http://www.cfr.org/healthmonitor.
  - This is a comprehensive resource that assess how well the international community is doing in addressing major threats, including global health. It includes an overview of the challenges, an interactive timeline of relief efforts, a directory of major organisations and key documents, and an interactive map showing critical countries.
- *WHO Factsheets.* http://www.who.int/topics.
  - Factsheets and key links on a wide range of global health and development topics.

Country information

- *CIA World Factbook.* http://www.cia.gov/library/publications/the-world-factbook.
  - Lists population, government, military and economic information for nations recognised by the United States. Good for background information on your destination country.
- *Global peace index.* http://www.visionofhumanity.org.
  - This project ranks 149 nations by their 'peacefulness', based on a basket of indicators.
- *WHO Country Profiles.* http://www.who.int/gho/countries.
  - Contains vital health information from the Global Health Observatory for each WHO member state, including mortality and burden of disease, outbreaks, immunisation profile, and health financing and workforce.

Emergency relief

- Anderson MB (1999). *Do Not Harm: How Aid Can Support Peace—or War.* Boulder: Lynne Rienner Publishers.
  - A practical guide for humanitarian health workers.
- Oxfam (2000). *Sphere Project (2011). The Sphere Project: Humanitarian Charter and Minimum Standards in Humanitarian Response.* http://www.sphereproject.org/.
- *Managing the Stress of Humanitarian Emergencies: A UNHCR Manual.* http://www.the-ecentre.net/resources/e_library/doc/managingstress.pdf.
  - Focuses on crisis situations, but contains useful advice for all overseas contexts where personal stress might arise.
- Walker P, Russ C (2010). *Professionalising the Humanitarian Sector: A Scoping Study. Enhancing Learning and Research for Humanitarian Assistance (ELRHA) Network.* http://www.elrha.org/professionalisation.

Health links

- Gedde M (2009). *The International Health Links Manual*, 2nd edition. Available for download at http://www.thet.org.uk or purchase at cpibookdelivery.
- Gordon M, Potts C (2008). *What Difference Are We Making? A Toolkit on Monitoring and Evaluation for Health Links*. Available for download at http://www.thet.org.uk or purchase at cpibookdelivery.
- http://www.thet.org/health-links/resources-for-links/.

Donating equipment overseas

- Imaging in LMIC Special Interest Group of the Society and College of Radiographers. http://www.idcsig.org/page6.html.
  - Advice on donating equipment overseas.
- THET. http://thet.org/wp-content/uploads/2009/10/makingdonations.pdf.

Travel health

- The National Travel Health Network and Centre (NaTHNaC). http://www.nathnac.org.
  - Provides health information for both health professionals and travellers. It also gives information on health risks in individual countries and disease outbreak reports around the globe.
- NaTHNaC (2010). *The 'Yellow Book': Health Information for Overseas Travel*. http://www.nathnac.org.

Pensions

- *Appendix II: NHS Pension Scheme—Further Advice*. http://www.dh.gov.uk/en/publicationsandstatistics/.

Tax and national insurance

- *Residents and Non-Residents Liability to Tax in the UK*. Booklet IR20. http://www.hmrc.gov.uk.
- *Social Security Abroad*. HMRC leaflet NI38. http://www.hmrc.gov.uk.

Personal accounts

- Fink SL (2004). *War Hospital: A True Story of Surgery and Survival*. New York: PublicAffairs.
  - The harrowing account of a group of young doctors who were trapped inside Srebrenica during the 1992 war.

- French Blaker L (2007). *Heart of Darfur*. London: Hodder and Stoughton.
  - New Zealand nurse's experiences from MSF posting in South Sudan.
- Orbinski J (2008). *An Imperfect Offering: Humanitarian Action in the Twenty-first Century*. Toronto: Doubleday Canada.
  - *Written by former head of MSF about his experiences in Rwanda and Somalia.*
- Pisani E (2008). *The Wisdom of Whores: Bureaucrats, Brothels, and the Business of AIDS*. New York: WW Norton.
  - Journalist-turned-epidemiologist writes about her work in the fast-evolving world of HIV/AIDS research and prevention in Africa and Asia.

General books

- Crisp N (2010). *Turning the World Upside Down: The Search for Global Health in the 21st Century*. London: Royal Society of Medicine.
  - Former head of the NHS outlines the reciprocal benefits for the UK and overseas of engaging in global health work.
- Easterly W (2007). *The White Man's Burden: Why the West's Efforts to Aid the Rest Have Done so Much Ill and so Little Good*. Oxford: Oxford University Press.
  - Alternative economist argues that aid is not the answer to poverty.
- Polman L (2010). *War Games: The Story of Aid and War in Modern Times*. New York: Viking.
  - This journalist argues, through colourful examples of her experiences in Africa and Asia, that humanitarian interventions prolong conflict.
- Sachs J (2005). *The End of Poverty: How We Can Make it Happen in Our Lifetime*. New York: Penguin.
  - Master economist outlines how aid is the answer to poverty.

Profession-specific information

- Thuman WD, Maxwell J (1992). *Where There Is no Doctor*, 2nd edition. Berkeley (CA): Hesperian.
  - This classic manual was primarily intended for village health workers; however, it is highly valued by clinicians in LMIC for its concise and practical information. It has been translated into over 100 languages. There are now several sister manuals, including *Where There Is no Psychiatrist* (see below).

Doctors

Medical students

- British Medical Association (2009). *Ethics and Medical Electives in Resource-Poor Countries—A Toolkit*. London: BMA.

- British Medical Association Medical Students Committee (2009). *Guidance on Planning an Elective at Home or Overseas*. London: BMA.
- Graham H (2005). *Beyond Borders: McGraw-Hill's Guide to Health Placements*. Columbus (OH): McGraw-Hill.
- Wilson M (2009). *The Medic's Guide to Work and Electives Around the World*, 3rd edition. London: Hodder Arnold.
  - http://www.medicstravel.co.uk is the accompanying website for the above book, where they also can organise your elective for you for a fee.

Trainees

- BMA International Department (2009). *Broadening Your Horizons: A Guide to Taking Time Out to Work and Train in Developing Countries*. http://www.bma.org.uk/international/working_abroad/broadeningyourhorizons.jsp
- Medical Speciality Training (England) (2010). *The Gold Guide: A Reference Guide for Postgraduate Specialty Training in the UK*. http://www.mmc.nhs.uk/specialty_training_2010/gold_guide.aspx.
  - Outlines how to request time out of programme, and what is required to progress as a speciality trainee.

RETIREES

- BMA (2010). *Advice for Retired Members on Volunteering and Global Health*. Available for members at http://www.bma.org.uk/international/working_abroad/.
- Christian Medical Fellowship (2008). *Re-tyred not Retired: Healthcare Mission in Later Life*. Order Reference Ret0805. London: Christian Medical Fellowship.
  - This booklet recounts the stories of eleven doctors who retired from professional work in the UK and found rewarding work overseas.

Speciality-specific information

ANAESTHETISTS

- Association of Anaesthetists of Great Britain and Northern Ireland (2002). *GAT Handbook on Organising a Year Abroad*. http://www.aagbi.org/pdf/gat_organising_year_abroad_2002.pdf.

GPS

- BMA (2008). *Guidance for GPs Taking Time Out of Employment to Work Overseas*. http://www.bma.org.uk/international/working_abroad.
  - This guidance is aimed at doctors working in general practice who want to take time out of employment to work or volunteer overseas, and then return to work as an NHS GP after the period of absence.

- Junior RCGP International Committee. http://www.jintc.org.
  - This is open to all UK GP trainees or GPs within 5 years of completing training. The Committee's objective is to facilitate the involvement of GP trainees and newly qualified GPs in educational international activities related to primary care. It also helps arrange international exchanges through the European Vasco da Gama Movement.

PAEDIATRICIANS
- RCPCH (2010). *VSO Fellowship Frequently Asked Questions.* http://www.rcpch.ac.uk/training/international-training-opportunities/voluntary-service-overseas.

GENERAL MEDICINE
- Parry E, Godfrey R, Mabey D, Gill G (eds) (2004). *Principles of Medicine in Africa*, 3rd edition. Cambridge: Cambridge University Press.

PSYCHIATRISTS
- Patel V (2003). *Where There Is no Psychiatrist: A Mental Health Care Manual.* London: Royal College of Psychiatrists.

Nurses and midwives

Students

- Christian Medical Fellowship (2004). *Preparing for Your Nursing or Midwifery Elective Overseas.* http://www.cmf.org.uk/internationalministries/electives.asp.
  - Written from a Christian perspective.
- RCM (2005). *For Student Midwives Undertaking Overseas Elective Experience: Frequently Asked Questions.* http://www.rcm.org.uk/college/students/.
- RCN (2008). *Overseas Electives for Nursing Students.* Available for members at http://www.rcn.org.uk/nursing/workingabroad.

Qualified

- RCM (2006). *Thinking About Working Abroad?* http://www.rcm.org.uk/college/international.
- RCN (2007). *Working with Humanitarian Organisations: A Guide for Nurses, Midwives and Healthcare Professionals.* Publication code 003 156. http://www.rcn.org.uk/nursing/workingabroad.
- RCN (2008). *General Information on Working Abroad.* http://www.rcn.org.uk/nursing/workingabroad.

- RCN (2008). *Guidelines for Members Experiencing Problems Whilst Working Overseas.* http://www.rcn.org.uk/nursing/workingabroad.
- RCN (2008). *Midwives Working Overseas.* http://www.rcn.org.uk/nursing/workingabroad.
- RCN International Humanitarian Community. Discussion forum and membership form. http://www.rcn.org.uk/development/communities/specialisms/international_humanitarian.
  - The RCN International Humanitarian Community brings together RCN members who have worked in, are currently working in or are interested in working in global health. It aims to provide a network for advice and support, and to raise the profile of international humanitarian work being undertaken by its members.

Dentists

- General Dental Council. *CPD for Dental Professionals Working Overseas.* http://www.gdc-uk.org/current+registrant/cpd+requirements.

Allied health professionals

- Hobbs L, McDonough S, O'Callaghan A (2002). *Life After injury: A Rehabilitation Manual for the Injured and Their Helpers.* Geneva: Third World Network.

Students

- Christian Medical Fellowship (2004). *Therapy Elective Overseas.* http://www.cmf.org.uk/internationalministries/electives.asp.
  - More a directory of useful information than specific advice. Written from a Christian perspective.

Qualified

HEALTH PROFESSIONS COUNCIL
- Health Professions Council (2006). *Your Guide to our Standards for CPD.* http://www.hpc-uk.org/registrants/cpd/.
- Health Professions Council (2008). *Returning to Practice.* http://www.hpc-uk.org/registrants/readmission.

SPEECH AND LANGUAGE THERAPISTS
- Communication Therapy International (2008). *Volunteer Advice Pack.* http://www.commtherapyint.com.

- Royal College of Speech and Language Therapists. *FAQs on Working Overseas*. Email: information@rcslt.org.

RADIOGRAPHERS

- Imaging in LMIC Special Interest Group of the Society and College of Radiographers. *Arranging an Overseas Radiography Placement/Elective*. http://www.idcsig.org/page6.html.

ORTHOPTISTS

- McNamara R (2010). *International Orthoptic Association Guidance for Orthoptists Considering Work in Developing Countries*. Available through British and Irish Orthoptic Society, email: bios@orthoptics.org.uk

Appendix 3

Useful courses

There are several courses available to prepare you for work overseas, from general introductions to year-long Masters. These can be a considerable investment in terms of time and money, so it's worth researching to find the right one for your learning needs. We highlight a selection of the most attended ones below—all prices were correct at the time of going to press.

Introductory courses

So You Think You Want to be a Relief Worker?

This is a popular 1-day course run by the charity RedR.

Where:	London
Aimed at:	Individuals from all backgrounds and professions who are considering working in the humanitarian sector
When:	Several times throughout the year
Duration:	1 day
Assessment:	Not assessed
Format:	Small group teaching
Cost:	£85 as individual
What you will gain:	"This course helps you to decide whether this is a career you want to pursue. You will hear first-hand experiences from relief workers, learn about the nature of humanitarian relief, and look at the skills you have to bring to the sector"
More info:	training@redr.org.uk, Tel. +44 (0)20 7840 6000

Crash Course in Overseas Medicine

Where:	Cheltenham General Hospital—Sandford Education Centre
Aimed at:	Doctors and senior nurses/midwives who are considering going to work in a developing country
When:	Yearly in May
Duration:	3 days
Assessment:	Not assessed
Format:	Seminars, hands-on practicals, small group teaching (limited to 20 delegates only)
Cost:	£315
What you will gain:	Practical advice, factual material, hands-on experience (not on patients), through hearing previous workers accounts a better understanding of how to prepare, where to go and what to do
More info:	alex.townsend@glos.nhs.uk, Tel. +44 (0)8454 224391

Short courses

Both RedR and the Institute of Health and International Development at the Queen Margaret University in Edinburgh offer an extensive programme of short courses for international health workers.

RedR areas include: health, planning and management; emergency preparedness; training and facilitation; safety and security; and humanitarian practice. See http://www.redr.org for more information.

Queen Margaret University areas include: human resources for health; international public health; sexual and reproductive health; and psychosocial interventions with displaced populations. See http://www.qmu.ac.uk/iihd/short_courses/short_cours-es.htm for more information.

Other popular courses are listed below.

CMF Developing Health Course

This provides high-quality training for work in resource-poor settings, covering a wide range of topics and practical skills. The course is aimed both at those currently working overseas who want to update their knowledge, and those who are planning to go who want to be equipped for the work they will do. In addition, many who are simply interested in international work have found it a useful opportunity to learn more about it and explore the possibilities of getting involved.

Where:	London
When:	Annually at the end of June
Duration:	2-week residential course (although you can choose to attend Special Interest Days only, or just one week of the course)
Aimed at:	Doctors, nurses and other allied health professionals
Assessment:	Not assessed
Format:	Lectures, practical skills workshops, group exercises, tutorials and case study analysis
Cost:	£950 (including accommodation and full board). Reduced rates are available for those currently working in resource-poor settings and for those attending less than the full fortnight
What you will gain:	Learn about the realities of work in a resource-poor setting. The course is usually approved for CPD by the Royal College of Physicians
More info:	

Infectious Diseases in Humanitarian Emergencies

This course is organised jointly with the WHO. The WHO also regularly runs this course outside the UK as 'Communicable Diseases in Humanitarian Emergencies'.

Where:	LSHTM
Aimed at:	"Those working in public health or related disciplines in LMIC, who have an interest and experience of infectious disease management in humanitarian emergencies and who would like to improve their skills or bring their knowledge up to date to support implementation of infectious disease projects/programmes in emergency settings"
When:	Yearly in April
Duration:	5 days
Assessment:	Not assessed, but letters of attendance provided
Format:	Mixture of lectures, cases studies, group exercises, discussions and practicals
Cost:	£375

➲

What you will gain:	"Day 1 will introduce concepts and epidemiological indicators, review infectious disease epidemiology, and conduct risk assessments and disease surveillance. Day 2 will cover outbreak investigation and response. Day 3 will cover infection control, social mobilisation, media and communication. Days 4–5 will cover the epidemiology of specific diseases (diarrhoeal diseases, acute respiratory infections, malaria, tuberculosis, HIV/AIDS, vaccine-preventable diseases such as measles and meningitis, pandemic influenza), and practical strategies for their prevention and control in emergencies"
More info:	*http://www.lshtm.ac.uk/prospectus/short/scidhe.htm*

Public Health in Crises and Transitional Contexts

Where:	London, Merlin offices
When:	Annually in July
Duration:	7 days full time
Aimed at:	Health professionals involved or interested in working in humanitarian relief
Assessment:	Not assessed
Format:	Lectures, group exercises, tutorials and case study analysis
Cost:	£600
What you will gain:	". . . understanding of acute and chronic health needs for populations affected by conflict, natural disasters, disease threat and health system collapse"
More info:	training@merlin.org.uk

Short Course in International Health Consultancy

This course is aimed at those who have the skills to take up consultancy or external advisor positions, but who would like more understanding of the process. Participants conduct a real-life consultancy during the course, and have the opportunity for a mentored consultancy project within 1 year of course completion.

Where:	Liverpool School of Tropical Medicine
When:	Annually in May
Duration:	3 weeks full time
Aimed at:	Health and development specialists with minimum 5 years' professional practice and ideally previous experience of short-term project work
Assessment:	Assessed
Format:	Lectures, group exercises, tutorials and case study analysis
Cost:	£2000
What you will gain:	". . . An opportunity to enhance and improve professional knowledge and skills in the provision and management of consultancy services within the context of global health"
More info:	http://www.lstmliverpool.ac.uk/learning_teaching/short_creds/international_health_consultancy.htm

Post-graduate certificate/diploma courses

Diploma in Tropical Medicine and Hygiene (DTM&H)

This course is offered by two institutes in the UK: LSTM and LSHTM.

The Diploma is recognised by the Royal College of Physicians and the Royal College of Paediatricians and Child Health as CPD (360 points). The Diploma is a requirement for UK doctors who want to specialise in tropical medicine. It also fulfils part of the requirements for the American Society of Tropical Medicine and Hygiene Certificate in Travel Medicine.

When:	Liverpool: Twice yearly (February–May and September–December). London: Once yearly (January–March)
Duration:	3 months full time
Aimed at:	Registered doctors, particularly those who have trained in medicine in a developed country but who intend to practise in the tropics
Format:	Lectures, seminars and practical sessions (very intensive)
Assessment:	Examination at end of course (multiple choice questions, essays and practical)
Cost:	Liverpool: £3,500 (includes examination fee) LSHTM: £4,750 (plus £195 examination fee)

➲

What you will gain:	"The course aims to teach doctors the skills required to understand, diagnose, treat and prevent diseases that are especially prevalent in tropical and LMIC where resources may be limited"
More info:	http://www.lshtm.ac.uk http://www.liv.ac.uk/lstm

Diploma in Tropical Nursing

Where:	LSHTM
Aimed at:	Registered nurses and midwives
When:	Twice yearly (September–February and March–July)
Duration:	One day per week (usually Wednesday) for 19 weeks
Assessment:	End of course examination (multiple choice questions and practical) Research-based essay on a relevant topic
Format:	Lectures and practical sessions
Cost:	£1,155
What you will gain:	"Knowledge of the causes, prevention and treatment of major tropical diseases, through lectures and practical laboratory sessions. Nurses and midwives should also gain an insight into primary health care in LMIC, learn to maximise care with minimum resources, and understand the importance of promoting health through prevention rather than cure"
More info:	http://www.lshtm.ac.uk/prospectus/short/stn.html

Diploma in the Medical Care of Catastrophes

This Diploma is prepared for by taking the 12-month part-time course in Conflict and Catastrophe Medicine run by the Society of Apothecaries of London.

Where:	London
Aimed at:	Civilian and military physicians, surgeons, dentists and nurses who will work as members of medical response teams
When:	One Saturday per month

➲

Duration:	January–December
Assessment:	Short-answer question paper Objective structured clinical and skills examination
Format:	Lectures and exercises
Cost:	£750
What you will gain:	"The Diploma is designed to demonstrate thorough specialist knowledge for those practitioners who are required to provide a medical and surgical response at the scene of major man-made and natural disasters. It is also intended to provide a means by which organisations can identify suitable personnel from those who volunteer to respond to such worldwide crises"
More info:	*http://www.apothecaries.org*

Masters degrees

Many of the masters programmes below are also offered at post-graduate certificate or diploma level, which require less module credits and are cheaper. For example, LSTM offers all its MSc courses including International Public Health, Humanitarian Health Programme Management, and Tropical Paediatrics at PG Cert/Dip level.

European Master in Disaster Medicine

This is a dedicated degree in disaster medicine delivered by several European and American institutions working together. It has a flexible structure consisting of online modular learning and then a residential course (usually in Europe).

Where:	Next residential course is in Italy
Aimed at:	All health professionals
When:	Start in February each year
Duration:	One academic year
Assessment:	Thesis and online examinations
Format:	Online distance learning modules 2-week residential course
Cost:	€4,000

What you will gain:	"During this program, you will develop analytical ability, strategic management knowledge, competence and problem-solving ability to deal with health problems in catastrophic events"
More info:	*http://www.dismedmaster.com*

Other Masters degree courses

The universities below offer a wide range of Masters degrees in various global health and tropical medicine topics. Most can be studied either on a full-time or part-time basis and some by distance learning.

- LSHTM (http://www.lshtm.ac.uk)
- LSTM (http://www.liv.ac.uk/lstm)
- UCL Institute for Global Health (http://www.ucl.ac.uk/global-health/)
- Nuffield Centre for International Health and Development (http://www.leeds.ac.uk/nuffield/)
- Institute of International Health and Development (http://www.qmu.ac.uk/iihd/)

Other courses

http://www.reliefweb.int is updated by the UN Office for the Coordination of Humanitarian Affairs, and includes information on many training courses for humanitarian workers.

Index

internet banking 171, 182
isolation 219

jetlag 199
job description, changes to 200
job listings 162–3

keeping up-to-date 246
knowledge transfer 40–1

lack of resources *see* resource-poor settings
languages 202–04
  additional 52
  English overseas 203
  essential phrases 204
  fluency in 94–6
  lack of knowledge of 30
  learning 72, 249
  number spoken 94
  teaching and training 232
  see also individual regions
laptop computers 192
late presentation 223–4
leadership 11
leading by example 255
leave of absence 178–9
  doctors in training 179
  NHS employees 178
life expectancy 7
lifestyle 31
links, international 290
living overseas 189–92
  communications 189–90
  personal items 190–2
  personal relationships 70–2, 190
LMIC *see* low and middle-income
    countries
local conditions 206
  contacts 248–9
  health priorities, distortion of 46–7
  staff
    attitude towards 43
    hierarchy 205, 221–2
local ownership of projects 260
LOCATE service 185
logframes 265
logistics 237
loneliness 206–07
long-term placements 67–8
low and middle-income countries 5, 12
low mood 275

malaria 6, 32
  chemoprophylaxis 100, 187–8

recurrence of 277
  transmission risk 101
Malawi, medical training 19
Maldives International Volunteer
    Programme 161
managers, overseas working 65
MDG *see* Millennium Development
    Goal
MDU *see* Medical Defence Union
measles, mortality reduction 7
Medair 159–60
Médecins sans Frontières 22, 137–40
Medical Defence Union 184
Medical and Dental Defence Union of
    Scotland 184
Medical Missions 163
Medical Officers 19
medical problems *see* health issues
medical products 11
Medical Protection Society 184
Medical Student Electives 157
  see also electives
medical students 54
  resources for 304
medical training 19
Medical Training Application Service 248
Medics Travel 158
medium-term placements 67
melatonin supplements 199
mentoring 179–80, 206, 243–4, 289–90
mercenaries 27
Mercy Ships 132–4, 284
Merlin (Medical Experts on the Frontline) 22,
    134–7
Middle East 108–09
midwives 58–61
  resources for 305–06
Millennium Development Goals 5, 9–10
misfits 27
Mission Finder 162
missionaries 27, 28–9
monetary issues 68
  electives 70
  income tax 69, 181–2
  National Insurance
    contributions 70, 181
  NHS pension contributions 69, 180
  salary 69
  student loan payments 181
  see also personal finances
money, access to abroad 182
monitoring and evaluation 264
  see also appraisal; mentoring
moral motivation 28